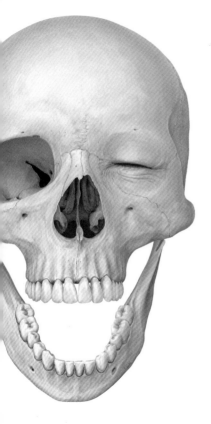

WinkingSkull.com *PLUS*

<u>Your</u> study aid for must-know microbi

T0265170

Register for WinkingSkull.com *PLUS* – master microbiology with this unique interactive online learning tool.

Use the access code below to register for **WinkingSkull.com *PLUS*** and view over 300 full-color illustrations from the book. The online content allows you to easily navigate by organ system or pathogen type. You can also view 16 animations with commentary that deepen understanding of the pathogens explored.

WinkingSkull.com *PLUS* has everything you need for course study and exam prep:

• More than 300 full-color illustrations

• Includes 16 richly animated videos with commentary

Simply visit Winking **instructions to get started today.**

If you do not already have a free WinkingSkull.com account, visit www.winkingskull.com, click on "Register" and complete the registration form. Enter the scratch-off code below.

If you already have a WinkingSkull.com account, go to the "Manage Account" page and click on the "Register a Code" link. Enter the scratch-off code below.

This product cannot be returned if the access code panel is scratched off.

Some functionalities on WinkingSkull.com require support for advanced web technologies. A major browser (IE, Chrome, Firefox, Safari) within the last three major versions is suggested for use on the site.

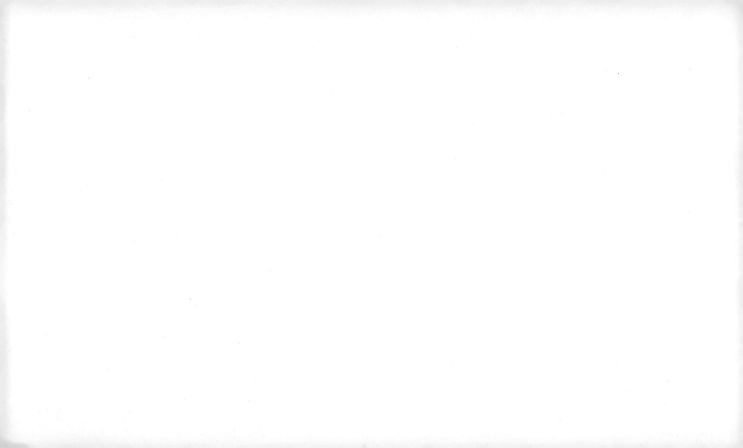

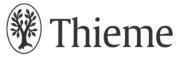

Microbiology in Your Pocket

Quick Pathogen Review

Melphine Harriott, PhD
Fellow, Clinical Microbiology
Department of Pathology, Microbiology and Immunology
Vanderbilt University Medical Center
Nashville, Tennessee, USA

313 illustrations

Thieme
New York · Stuttgart · Delhi · Rio de Janeiro

Acquisitions Editor: Delia K. DeTurris
Developmental Editor: Julia Nollen
Managing Editor: Torsten Scheihagen
Editorial Director, Educational Products: Anne M. Sydor, PhD
Director, Editorial Services: Mary Jo Casey
Production Editor: Barbara Chernow
International Production Director: Andreas Schabert
International Marketing Director: Fiona Henderson
International Sales Director: Louisa Turrell
Director of Sales, North America: Mike Roseman
Senior Vice President and Chief Operating Officer: Sarah Vanderbilt
President: Brian D. Scanlan
Typesetter: Carol Pierson, Chernow Editorial Associates, Inc.

Library of Congress Cataloging-in-Publication Data
Names: Harriott, Melphine, author.
Title: Microbiology in your pocket : quick pathogen review / Melphine Harriott.
Description: New York : Thieme, [2018]
Identifiers: LCCN 2017013563 (print) | LCCN 2017014708 (ebook) | ISBN 9781626234154 (alk. paper) |
    ISBN 9781626234161 (eISBN)
Subjects: | MESH: Bacterial Infections | Virus Diseases | Protozoan Infections | Virulence | Case Reports |
    Problems and Exercises
Classification: LCC RA644.B32 (ebook) | LCC RA644.B32 (print) | NLM WC 18.2 | DDC 614.5/7—dc23
LC record available at https://lccn.loc.gov/2017013563

Copyright © 2018 by Thieme Medical Publishers, Inc.

Thieme Publishers New York
333 Seventh Avenue, New York, NY 10001 USA
+1 800 782 3488, customerservice@thieme.com

Thieme Publishers Stuttgart
Rüdigerstrasse 14, 70469 Stuttgart, Germany
+49 [0]711 8931 421, customerservice@thieme.de

Thieme Publishers Delhi
A-12, Second Floor, Sector-2, Noida-201301
Uttar Pradesh, India
+91 120 45 566 00, customerservice@thieme.in

Thieme Publishers Rio de Janeiro, Thieme Publicações Ltda.
Edifício Rodolpho de Paoli, 25º andar
Av. Nilo Peçanha, 50 – Sala 2508
Rio de Janeiro 20020-906 Brasil
+55 21 3172-2297 / +55 21 3172-1896

Cover design: Thieme Publishing Group

Printed in China by Everbest Printing Co.   5 4 3 2 1

ISBN 978-1-62623-415-4

Also available as an e-book:
eISBN 978-1-62623-416-1

Important note: Medicine is an ever-changing science undergoing continual development. Research and clinical experience are continually expanding our knowledge, in particular our knowledge of proper treatment and drug therapy. Insofar as this book mentions any dosage or application, readers may rest assured that the authors, editors, and publishers have made every effort to ensure that such references are in accordance with **the state of knowledge at the time of production of the book.**

Nevertheless, this does not involve, imply, or express any guarantee or responsibility on the part of the publishers in respect to any dosage instructions and forms of applications stated in the book. **Every user is requested to examine carefully** the manufacturers' leaflets accompanying each drug and to check, if necessary in consultation with a physician or specialist, whether the dosage schedules mentioned therein or the contraindications stated by the manufacturers differ from the statements made in the present book. Such examination is particularly important with drugs that are either rarely used or have been newly released on the market. Every dosage schedule or every form of application used is entirely at the user's own risk and responsibility. The authors and publishers request every user to report to the publishers any discrepancies or inaccuracies noticed. If errors in this work are found after publication, errata will be posted at www.thieme.com on the product description page.

Some of the product names, patents, and registered designs referred to in this book are in fact registered trademarks or proprietary names even though specific reference to this fact is not always made in the text. Therefore, the appearance of a name without designation as proprietary is not to be construed as a representation by the publisher that it is in the public domain.

www.fsc.org

100%

Paper from well-managed forests

FSC® C124385

This work is dedicated to all my past and future students who motivate me to be better and to learn more.

I am indebted to my husband, Alwyn, and my parents Melchizedek and Josephine
for their encouragement and support during the development of this project.

Contents

Preface

Microbiology in Your Pocket: Quick Pathogen Review is a collection of notecards intended to aid medical students, physician assistant students, dental students, and other graduate health science students while studying for a medical microbiology course. These cards can also be utilized as a supplemental study tool for the preparation of United States Medical Licensing Examination (USMLE) Step 1, Comprehensive Osteopathic Medical Licensing Examination (COMLEX) Level 1, Physician Assistant National Certifying Exam (PANCE) and National Board Dental Examination (NBDE).

The cards contain high-yield information that encompasses many of the clinically significant bacteria, viruses, yeast, and parasites that are covered in a graduate level medical microbiology course or on a board exam. It was not feasible to cover all clinically relevant microorganisms or all pertinent information regarding each microbe in this succinct review, hence students should use this as a supplement rather than the sole source in preparation for a course or board examination.

The cards are color coded by pathogen type using the following color scheme:

Pink: Gram-negative bacteria
Purple: Gram-positive bacteria
Gray: Organisms that do not Gram stain or Gram stain poorly
Green: Viruses
Blue: Fungi
Orange: Parasites

Each pathogen/card is assigned a primary organ system when possible and cards are organized by this primary organ system assignment. Primary organ systems include:

Nervous System
Head and Neck
Respiratory System
Blood/Lymph/Systemic Infections
Gastrointestinal System
Liver and Biliary System
Renal and Urinary Systems
Reproductive System
Skin, Soft Tissue, and Musculoskeletal Systems

However, note that it is not possible to assign a primary organ system to some pathogens since they may infect multiple anatomic sites. Hence, these pathogens are in a chapter designated Multiple Organ Systems.

Each card contains similar information. The various sections of each card are explained in further detail below:

Micro gem: The front of some cards contains a "Micro gem" which is small bit of free-standing information that is pertinent to the microorganism presented on the card.

Vignette(s): The front of each card contains one or more clinical vignettes. An explanation for each vignette is on the back of the same card.

Images: Most cards contain images such as microscopic images of the pathogen, biochemical tests or clinical images of infections with the pathogen. Note that although the images are on the front of the card are numbered and appear under the vignette, the images are are linked to concepts found on the back of the card.

The back of each card contains the following:

Description: For bacteria, this section includes Gram stain reaction/morphology and other descriptive features of the organism. For viruses, this includes the viral taxonomy and a description of the genetic nature of the virus. For fungi, this section includes a microscopic description of the characteristic features of the fungi. Lastly, for parasites, the taxonomy, alternative name as well the microscopic features of the parasite are listed in this section.

Infections: As previously mentioned, when possible organisms were assigned a primary organ system based on the chief infectious disease associated with that pathogen. Other infections that may be less common are listed under the heading "Other". Note that this section does not contain a comprehensive list of all the potential infections associated with a pathogen, but rather the most common conditions.

Pathogenesis: Most cards will have a pathogenesis/virulence mechanism, such as toxin production, listed in this section.

Epidemiology: Each card contains epidemiological information including transmission and groups that are at high risk for infections with that pathogen.

Diagnosis: Each card has select microbiologic diagnostic tests that may be used to identify the organism. Note this is not a comprehensive list and actual diagnostic testing may vary based on the clinical situation.

Prevention: Some cards have examples of prevention methods, such as immunization, listed in this section.

Treatment: Each card contains examples of effective antimicrobials for the pathogen. This information should not be utilized for actual clinical treatment as many factors must be considered when making decisions regarding antimicrobial therapy.

Animation(s): Some cards contain animations that provide a more detailed explanation of the pathogenesis mechanism. These animations may be accessed via WinkingSkull.com; please see the scratch-off page on the inside front cover for instructions on how to access the site.

Explanation: Each card contains explanations for the vignettes which are on the front of the card.

Cross-references: To assist students in making correlations between organisms and/or infections, some cards contain cross-references to other cards. These cross-references include the number of the card, which will enable readers to locate them.

There are also cross-references to indicate a similarity between organisms. For example within the Diagnosis section of the *Listeria monocytogenes* card, note the cross-reference to *Streptococcus agalactiae* which is indicated in the following manner: CAMP test positive with block head hemolysis (2). *See also* ● 5, *Streptococcus agalactiae* ●. Both organisms are CAMP test positive and students may refer to the *S. agalactiae* (which is Gram positive as indicated by the purple dots) card for further details.

Appendix: The appendix contains tables, line art, and graphs that summarize information presented throughout the cards.

Melphine Harriott, PhD

Acknowledgments

I am extremely grateful for the following students who assisted me in the development of *Microbiology in Your Pocket: Quick Pathogen Review*:

Joshua McCarron—Joshua assisted in the development of the initial version of the notecards while a second-year medical student at Oakland University William Beaumont School of Medicine. He is now completing an internal medicine residency at Wright State University / Wright-Patterson Air Force Base.

Erik Sweet—Erik developed the initial web-based version of the notecards during his first year at Oakland University William Beaumont School of Medicine. He is now an ophthalmology resident at the University of Michigan.

Paige Peterson and Lauren McNickle—assisted in modifying and editing the original notecards. Without their hard work, this project would have not been completed in a timely manner. Both Paige and Lauren worked on this project during their fourth year at Frank H. Netter MD School of Medicine / Quinnipiac University. Paige and Lauren were fourth and third year medical students respectively at the Frank H Netter MD School of Medicine/Quinnipiac University while working on this project. Paige will soon be starting the Anatomic and Clinical Pathology Residency Program at the University of Colorado.

This work was completed in part while the author had the following affiliations:

Assistant Professor
Midwestern University
Chicago College of Osteopathic Medicine
Downers Grove, Illinois, USA

Assistant Professor
Oakland University
William Beaumont School of Medicine
Rochester, Michigan, USA

Abbreviations

ACh	acetylcholine		HIV	human immunodeficiency virus
ADP	adenosine diphosphate ribose		IL	interleukin
AFB	acid-fast bacilli		INF	interferon
AIDS	acquired immunodeficiency syndrome		GABA	gamma aminobutyric acid
ALT	alanine amino transferase		GI	gastrointestinal
AST	aspartate amino transferase		GNC	gram-negative cocci
ATP	adenosine triphosphate		GNR	gram-negative rod
cGMP	cyclic GMP		GPC	gram-positive cocci
CAMP	Christie-Atkins-Munch-Peterson		GPR	gram-positive rod
cAMP	cyclic adenosine monophosphate		HIV	human immunodeficiency virus
CBC	complete blood count		IV	intravenous
CDC	Centers for Disease Control		IVDU	intravenous drug use
CFU	colony forming unit		KOH	potassium hydroxide
cGMP	cyclic guanosine monophosphate		LPS	lipopolysaccharide
CO2	carbon dioxide		MAP	mitogen-activated protein
COPD	chronic obstructive pulmonary disease		MCV	mean corpuscular volume
CSF	cerebrospinal fluid		MHC	major histocompatibility complex
CT	computed tomography		MRI	magnetic resonance imaging
DIC	disseminated intravascular coagulation		O&P	ova and parasite
DFA	direct fluorescent antibody		PCR	polymerase chain reaction
EAEC	enteroaggregative *Escherichia coli*		PMNs	polymorphonuclear cell
EAST	enteroaggregative heat stable toxin		RBC	red blood cell
EHEC	enterohemorrhagic *Escherichia coli*		SNARE	soluble attachment protein receptor
EPEC	enteropathogenic *Escherichia coli*		STEC	shiga-toxin producing *E. coli*
EIA	enzyme immunoassay		TNF	tumor necrosis factor
EIEC	enteroinvasive *Escherichia coli*		U.S.	United States
ELISA	enzyme linked immunosorbent assay		UTIs	urinary tract infections
ETEC	enterotoxigenic *Escherichia coli*		WBC	white blood cell

Micro gem: Both *Clostridium* and *Bacillus* are gram-positive rods with spores. *Clostridium* are anaerobic, whereas *Bacillus* are aerobic.

See also ● 63, *Clostridium difficile* ●; ● 110, *Clostridium perfringens* ●; ● 2, *Clostridium tetani* ●; ● 109, *Bacillus anthracis* ●; ● 61, *Bacillus cereus* ●

Vignette 1: A 42-year-old woman presents to the emergency department with nausea, vomiting, abdominal pain, and diarrhea of 24 hours' duration. Her husband sought medical assistance for her when he noticed she was experiencing dry mouth, difficulty with her vision, and weakness in her arms. The husband states that his wife recently consumed home-canned peaches.

Vignette 2: A 4-month-old infant presents to the emergency department with decreased movement. The parents state that the child has been irritable, drooling, and not feeding well for the past 3 days. The child is breast-fed, and the mother states that she noticed a decreased ability to suck and that the baby's cry seems "weak" and "not normal." On examination, the child has noticeable hypotonia, with poor head control and is dehydrated. The child's temperature at the time of examination is 37.2°C (99°C). The cerebrospinal fluid analysis is unremarkable.

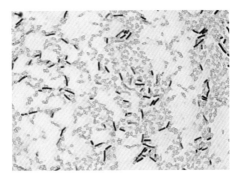

(1)

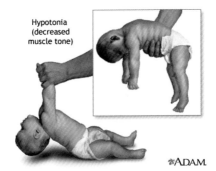

Hypotonia (decreased muscle tone)

✳A.D.A.M.

(2) *Source:* National Institutes of Health (https://www.nlm. nih.gov/medlineplus/ency/imagepages/17229.htm)

1 *Clostridium botulinum*

DESCRIPTION
Gram-positive rods, large, boxcar shaped (1)
Spore-producer (1)
Obligate anaerobe

INFECTIONS
PRIMARY
Botulism
Nervous
  Foodborne adult botulism: 12- to 36-hour incubation; fixed or dilated pupils, diplopia, difficulty swallowing, dry mouth, and descending paralysis (limp/flaccid muscles)
  Infant botulism/floppy baby syndrome (2): hypotonia

OTHER
Skin and soft tissue: wound botulism

PATHOGENESIS
Exotoxin/neurotoxin: botulinum toxin types A–G: heat-labile protease that cleaves SNAREs and prevents ACh release at neuromuscular junction

EPIDEMIOLOGY
Spores found in soil
Transmission: Foodborne adult botulism: ingestion of preformed toxin in food—commonly associated foods include smoked, vacuum-packed and alkaline home-canned foods
  Infant botulism: most likely inhalation of spores that colonize GI tract and produce toxin *in vivo* (in the past mainly attributed to ingestion and was commonly associated with honey and powdered formula)
  Wound botulism: bacteria infects wound, then forms toxin *in vivo*

DIAGNOSIS
Toxin detection
  Foodborne adult botulism: serum (preferred), stool or vomitus
  Infant botulism: stool
  Wound: pus or tissue from wound site

TREATMENT
Antimicrobials not proven effective
However, penicillin G, metronidazole may be used
Aminoglycosides are not typically used because they enhance the neuromuscular blockade caused by the toxin
Antitoxin
  Equine derived—for adults only
  Human-derived immunoglobulin (baby immunoglobulin [BabyBIG] or BIG-IV)—for infants < 1-year-old

ANIMATION
http://go.thieme.com/microb/Video1.1

Explanation 1: *Clostridium botulinum* is an anaerobic gram-positive rod with spores. This pathogen may cause wound infections, infant botulism, or foodborne infections, such as in this case. Adult foodborne botulism is associated with canned foods, including vegetables, fruit, and fish. The classic presentation is dry mouth and descending weakness. This is due to the botulinum toxin that inhibits release of acetylcholine.

Explanation 2: *Clostridium botulinum* is an anaerobic gram-positive rod with spores. This pathogen may cause wound infections, foodborne infections, or infant botulism, such as in this case. In the past, infant botulism was associated with honey, but recently it is thought that infections arise from inhalation of spores that may be found in the soil and dusty environments. The classic presentation of infant botulism is a "floppy" baby (i.e., hypotonia). Unlike adults, infants especially from birth to 12 months do not have the appropriate immune response and intestinal flora to prevent infections with this organism, especially if the inoculum concentration is high. The botulinum toxin inhibits release of acetylcholine.

Micro gem: The tetanus toxin inhibits inhibitory neurotransmitters, GABA and glycine, while the botulinum toxin inhibits the excitatory neurotransmitter, ACh.

See also ● 1, *Clostridium botulinum* ●

Vignette: A 58-year-old homeless man is brought to the emergency department by the police, who have found him under the influence of drugs and alcohol, missing shoes and socks, and barely responsive. Upon examination his temperature is 40.1°C (104°F), his heart rate is 90 beats/min, and his blood pressure is 60/40 mm Hg. In addition, he is having difficulty breathing, and his neck is stiff and hyperextended. Trismus and opisthotonic posturing are also noted. His feet are obviously gangrenous and ulcerated.

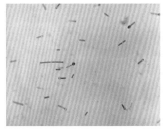

(1) *Source:* CDC/Dr. Lillian V. Holdeman CDC public health library PHIL (phil.cdc. gov) image No. 12056 (http://phil.cdc.gov/phil/details_linked. asp?pid=12056)

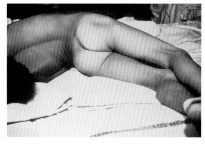

(2) *Source:* CDC public health library PHIL (phil.cdc.gov) image No. 6373 (http://phil.cdc.gov/phil/details_linked.asp?pid=6373)

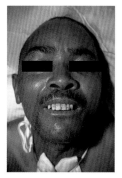

(3) *Source:* CDC/Dr. Thomas F. Sellers/Emory University CDC public health library PHIL (phil.cdc.gov) image No. 2857 (http://phil.cdc.gov/phil/ details_linked.asp?pid= 2857)

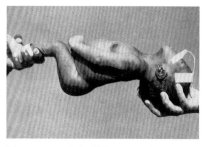

(4) *Source:* CDC public health library PHIL (phil.cdc.gov) image No. 6374 (http://phil.cdc.gov/phil/details_linked.asp?pid=6374)

2   *Clostridium tetani*

DESCRIPTION
Gram-positive rods (1), large, boxcar shaped
Spore-producer
Obligate anaerobe

INFECTIONS
PRIMARY
Tetanus
Nervous: tetanus—generalized tetanus (2,3); results in muscle rigidity/spastic paralysis with trismus (lockjaw) and risus sardonicus (grinning expression resulting from facial muscle spasm)

OTHER
Head and neck: localized tetanus
Neonatal (rare): neonatal tetanus (4)

PATHOGENESIS
Exotoxin/neurotoxin: tetanospasmin—protease that cleaves SNAREs and prevents release of GABA and/or glycine at alpha motor neuron
Binds to end of motor neurons and is transported in a retrograde manner to nervous system

EPIDEMIOLOGY
Spores found in the soil
Transmission:
Direct contact with spores—most often after trauma to skin
Neonatal—associated with umbilical cord contamination at delivery

DIAGNOSIS
Usually made on clinical findings

PREVENTION
Vaccine: toxoid vaccines—DTaP, DT, Td, Tdap
Boosters required

TREATMENT
Antimicrobial: to target bacteria
Effective antimicrobial agents include metronidazole and penicillin
Human tetanus immune globulin (HTIG): to target unbound toxin
HTIG can only bind and remove toxin that has not yet bound to a nerve ending.

ANIMATION
http://go.thieme.com/microb/Video2.1

Explanation: This man has tetanus which is caused by *Clostridium tetani*. This pathogen is an anaerobic gram-positive rod with spores. It produces a toxin that prevents neurons from releasing GABA and glycine. The symptoms described in this case are classic symptoms observed with tetanus. The lack of shoes and socks provides a route of transmission for spores, which are found in soil.

3   *Listeria monocytogenes*

Micro gem: The most common bacterial agents of neonatal meningitis are *Listeria monocytogenes*, ● 5, *Streptococcus agalactiae* ●, and ● 129, *Escherichia coli* K1 ●

Vignette: A 45-year-old woman presents to the emergency department with ataxia and tremors. She states that a few days prior she had experienced a severe headache, fever, and stiff neck. In addition, she has recently been diagnosed with acute myeloid leukemia and is currently undergoing treatment. She mentions that she lives on a goat farm and makes and sells homemade cheese. Her temperature is 38.4°C (101.1°F). CSF analysis demonstrates low glucose, elevated protein, and elevated neutrophils. A Gram stain from the CSF shows gram-positive rods.

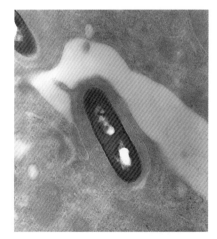

(1) *Source:* CDC/Dr. Balasubr Swaminathan; Peggy Hayes
   CDC public health library PHIL (phil.cdc.gov) image
   No. 10828
   (http://cdc.gov/phil/details_linked.asp?pid=10828)

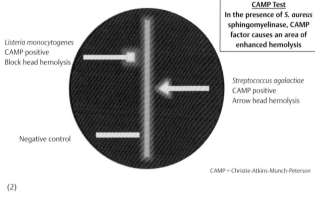

Listeria monocytogenes
CAMP positive
Block head hemolysis

Streptococcus agalactiae
CAMP positive
Arrow head hemolysis

Negative control

CAMP Test
In the presence of *S. aureus* sphingomyelinase, CAMP factor causes an area of enhanced hemolysis

CAMP = Christie-Atkins-Munch-Peterson

(2)

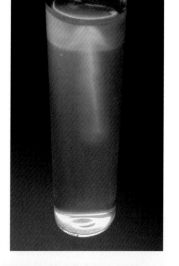

(3)

3 Listeria monocytogenes

DESCRIPTION Short gram-positive rods or coccobacilli (1)

INFECTIONS
PRIMARY

Gastrointestinal: gastroenteritis—diarrhea
Nervous: meningitis, meningoencephalitis
Systemic: bacteremia; during pregnancy, infections manifest as febrile "flu-like" illness which can cause spontaneous abortions/fetal death
Neonatal: meningitis
Congenital: granulomatosis infantiseptica

PATHOGENESIS

Facultative intracellular pathogen
Exotoxin/cytotoxin: listeriolysin O (LLO)—assists with intracellular survival and escape
actA: used to create actin tail; propels itself through cell cytoplasm by assembly of this actin tail. *See also* ● 71, *Shigella* ●

EPIDEMIOLOGY

Transmission:
  Post-natal infections: foodborne—commonly associated foods include soft cheese, unpasteurized milk, cold deli meats, ice cream, fruits, vegetables
  Congenital and neonatal: vertical (*in utero* or perinatal)
Mild infections in immunocompetent
High risk for meningitis:
  Neonates
  Elderly
  Individuals with decreased cell-mediated immunity

DIAGNOSIS

Culture: beta-hemolytic, catalase positive, growth in cold (4°C), CAMP test positive with block-head hemolysis (2). *See also* ● 5, *Streptococcus agalactiae* ●
Motility: tumbling on wet preparation or umbrella-shaped in semi-solid media (3) at room temperature (25°C)

TREATMENT

Depends on age, immune status: meningitis/meningoencephalitis
Ampicillin plus gentamicin

ANIMATION http://go.thieme.com/microb/Video3.1

Explanation: *Listeria monocytogenes* is a facultative intracellular gram-positive rod. Infections are transmitted from contaminated food and unlike most pathogenic organisms, *Listeria* can endure cold temperatures, which allows it to survive refrigeration. In immunocompetent individuals, infections are asymptomatic or manifest as mild gastroenteritis. However in neonates, the elderly and immunocompromised individuals meningitis may occur. This organism has several mechanisms of pathogenesis including production of exotoxins, invasion of host cells, intracellular survival, and propulsion from cell-to-cell within the host.

4 *Neisseria meningitidis*

Micro gem: Splenic macrophages facilitate opsonization and phagocytosis of encapsulated bacteria. Therefore, asplenic individuals are at increased risk for infections with pathogens containing polysaccharide capsules including *Neisseria meningitidis*, ● 136, *Streptococcus pneumoniae* ●, and ● 130, *Haemophilus influenzae* ●.

Vignette: A 19-year-old male college student presents to the emergency department with a fever and lethargy. His roommate states he appeared normal the evening before but had complained of a severe headache. That morning the roommate found him in bed moaning and complaining of drowsiness and neck pain. At the time of examination his temperature is 40.3°C (104.5°F). In addition, nuchal rigidity and a purpuric rash on his legs and trunk are noted. A lumbar puncture demonstrates decreased CSF glucose, elevated CSF protein, and elevated CSF white blood cells, particularly neutrophils. The CSF Gram stain demonstrates the presence of gram-negative diplococci.

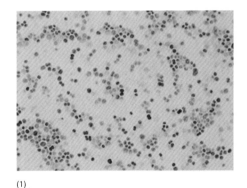

(1)

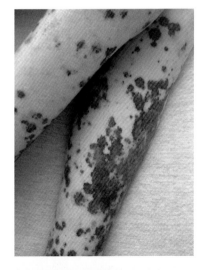

(2) *Source:* Petechial rash, User: DrFO.Jr.Tn (own work) [CC BY-SA 3.0 (http://creativecommons.org/licenses/by-sa/3.0)], via Wikimedia Commons (https://commons.wikimedia.org/wiki/File:Petechial_rash.JPG)

4   *Neisseria meningitidis*

DESCRIPTION   Gram-negative diplococci, kidney/coffee bean-shaped (1)
Clinically significant serogroups include A, B, C, X, Y, Z, W135, and L
Alternative name: meningococcus (MC)

INFECTIONS
PRIMARY

Nervous: meningitis with or without meningococcemia
Systemic: meningococcemia; DIC and petechial rash may occur (2); severe infection associated with Waterhouse-Friderichsen syndrome

PATHOGENESIS   Capsule
Endotoxin/lipooligosaccharide (LOS): similar function as LPS
Pili: capable of phase and antigenic variation
Outer membrane proteins: opacity (opa) proteins—assist in adhesion—capable of phase and antigenic variation
IgA protease: destroys IgA
   See also ● 105, *Neisseria gonorrhoeae* ●; ● 130, *Haemophilus influenzae* ●; ● 136, *Streptococcus pneumoniae* ●

EPIDEMIOLOGY   Transmission: respiratory droplets
High risk:
   Children and young adults
   Individuals living in close quarters, such as college and military campuses
   Individuals with complement deficiency (C5–C9)
   Asplenic individuals

PREVENTION   Vaccine: currently available for A, B, C, W, and Y serogroups
   Conjugate vaccine: infants, children, and adults
   Polysaccharide vaccine: older adults/elderly
   Recombinant vaccine (for serogroup B only): young adults

DIAGNOSIS   Culture: fastidious, best growth on chocolate or selective media such as Thayer-Martin. *See also* ● 105, *Neisseria gonorrhoeae* ●
PCR from CSF
Latex agglutination for capsular serogroup

TREATMENT   Ceftriaxone

ANIMATION   http://go.thieme.com/microb/Video4.1; http://go.thieme.com/microb/Video4.2

Explanation: This man has meningitis caused by *Neisseria meningitidis*. Populations in close quarters, such as on college campuses and military bases, are at a higher risk for meningitis with this organism. *N. meningitidis* is a gram-negative diplococcus and is often referred to as meningococcus. The main mechanism of virulence is a capsule. Meningitis may be present in conjunction with meningococcemia. Alternatively, meningitis or meningococcemia may be present independent of one another. The petechial rash is a classic sign of infection of the organism, but note that the rash is not always present. CSF findings of decreased glucose, elevated protein, and elevated neutrophils are consistent with bacterial infection.

Vignette: A 1-day-old infant develops a fever, poor feeding, and irritability. The baby was born full-term via vaginal delivery. His temperature is 38.2°C (100.8°F) and his blood pressure is 90/42 mmHg. Physical examination shows a bulging fontanelle and nuchal rigidity. A CSF Gram stain demonstrates gram-positive cocci in chains.

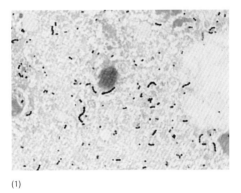

(1)

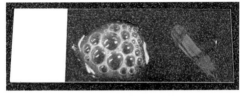

(2)

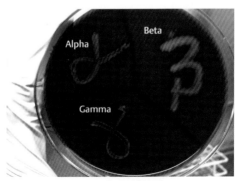

(3)

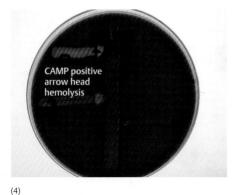

(4)

5 Streptococcus agalactiae

DESCRIPTION

Gram-positive cocci in chains (1)
Alternative name: group B streptococcus (GBS)

INFECTIONS

PRIMARY

Congenital/neonatal
    Nervous: meningitis
    Respiratory: pneumonia
    Systemic: bacteremia, sepsis

OTHER

Pregnant females
    Renal/urinary: UTIs
    Reproductive: chorioamnionitis, postpartum endometritis
Non-pregnant adults
    Skin and soft tissue/musculoskeletal: cellulitis, ulcers, wounds, arthritis, osteomyelitis
    Systemic: bacteremia

PATHOGENESIS

Capsule

EPIDEMIOLOGY

May colonize gastrointestinal, genitourinary, or upper respiratory tract
Transmission:
    Displacement of endogenous strains
    Congenital/neonatal: vertical (perinatal)

DIAGNOSIS

Culture: catalase negative (2), beta-hemolytic (3), CAMP test positive—arrow head hemolysis (4). *See also* ● 3, *Listeria monocytogenes* ●
PCR from rectal/vaginal swabs—used mainly for prenatal screening

PREVENTION

Vaginal cultures are obtained from pregnant women at 35 to 37 weeks' gestation, and if GBS positive, IV antimicrobials are administered during delivery

TREATMENT

Penicillin G

Explanation: The three main bacterial pathogens that cause meningitis in newborns are *Streptococcus agalactiae,* ● 129, *Escherichia coli* ●, and ● 3, *Listeria monocytogenes* ●. Of these, only *S. agalactiae* is a gram-positive coccus in chains. Some pregnant women carry GBS in their GI tract or vagina, and can transmit the pathogen to the infant during parturition. Infections in newborns may be early onset (within 24 hours of birth) or late onset (4–5 weeks after birth) and include not only meningitis but pneumonia and sepsis as well.

6 Bunyavirus

Micro gem: Most bunyaviruses are **ar**thropod **bo**rne flavivirus (**arbo**viruses)

Arbovirus is not a true taxonomic classification. Instead, it encompasses viruses from multiple families.

See also ● 10, *Alphavirus* ●; ● 49, Colorado tick virus ●

Vignette: A 4-year-old boy from Wisconsin returns from a week-long summer camping trip with his family with a fever. The following day he is still febrile and is now vomiting and also complains of a headache. His mother manages his symptoms with an analgesic and sends the boy to bed. The next day, the boy is lethargic and still febrile, so the mother takes him to emergency department. While there the boy has a seizure. His temperature is 39°C (102.2°F). Physical exam is remarkable for Babinski's sign. The boy's legs and arms contain several mosquito bites. A lumbar puncture is performed, and glucose is normal and protein is slightly elevated. The CSF Gram stain shows many mononuclear cells but no bacteria present. Serological analysis confirms the diagnosis.

6 Bunyavirus

DESCRIPTION
Taxonomy: Bunyavirus family
Virus properties: single-stranded, negative-sense RNA, enveloped, segmented genome
Clinically significant viruses (not a complete list):
  Arbovirus: California serogroup viruses—California encephalitis virus (CEV) and LaCrosse virus (LV)
  Hantavirus—which is not an arbovirus

INFECTIONS
PRIMARY
CEV and LV
  Nervous: meningoencephalitis, encephalitis
Hantavirus
  Systemic and respiratory: febrile illness followed by cardiopulmonary symptoms, hemorrhagic fever may occur

EPIDEMIOLOGY
CEV and LV
  Transmission/vector: bite of a mosquito
  Reservoir: rodents
  Geographic distribution: North America
Hantavirus
  Transmission: inhalation of contaminated aerosols from rodent (usually mice or rats) excreta
  Geographic distribution: North and South America

DIAGNOSIS
Serology: antibody testing
PCR

TREATMENT
Supportive

Explanation: This boy has encephalitis caused by LaCrosse virus. This pathogen is part of the California serogroup viruses and part of the Bunyavirus family. Infections are transmitted via the bite of a mosquito. This infection may be seen in many regions of North and South America, but several cases have been recorded in the Midwest. Infections may be asymptomatic or present as encephalitis. Children are more likely to present with signs and symptoms of encephalitis, whereas adults tend be asymptomatic. The CSF may show elevated monocytic cells; however, no organisms will be seen with a Gram stain because this pathogen is a virus. Serological or molecular testing is necessary to confirm the diagnosis.

7 Arthropod Borne Flaviviruses

Micro gem: Most flaviviruses are **ar**thropod **bo**rne viruses (**arbo**viruses)

Arbovirus is not a true taxonomic classification. Instead, it encompasses viruses from multiple families.

Hepatitis C virus is a flavivirus but is NOT arthropod borne

See also ● 91, Hepatitis C virus ●; ● 10, *Alphavirus* ●; ● 6, Bunyavirus ●

Vignette: A 35-year-old woman travels from the United States to Thailand to visit her family. She stays for a month. Within 3 days of her return to the United States, she experiences a sudden onset of fever, chills, malaise, and headache. After 3 days of these symptoms, she visits the emergency department. In addition to her initial symptoms, she is now also experiencing joint and muscle pain. When questioned, she pinpoints her headache as severe pain behind her eye. Her temperature is 39.9°C (103.8°F). She is ill appearing, and a small, red macular rash is seen on her face and neck. WBCs, platelets, and sodium levels are decreased. Serology and reverse-transcriptase PCR confirms the causative agent.

7 Arthropod Borne Flaviviruses

DESCRIPTION
Taxonomy: Flavivirus family
Virus properties: single-stranded, positive-sense RNA, enveloped
Clinically significant viruses: Dengue, Japanese encephalitis, St. Louis encephalitis, West Nile, Yellow fever, Zika

Virus	Primary Infection	Epidemiology			Diagnosis
		Transmission/Vector	Reservoir	Geographic Distribution	
Dengue	Asymptomatic or systemic: • Febrile illness with constitutional symptoms, myalgia, arthralgia, retro-orbital pain, and scarlatiniform rash • Hemorrhagic fever and shock may occur with some strains	Bite of mosquito (*Aedes aegypti* and *Aedes albopictus*) Vertical: usually *in utero*	Primates	Tropical regions; Asia, Central and South America	Serology: antibody testing PCR
Japanese encephalitis	Nervous: encephalitis	Bite of mosquito	Pigs, birds	Southeast and South Asia	Serology: antibody testing PCR
St. Louis encephalitis			Birds	North America and parts of South America	
West Nile	Asymptomatic or systemic: febrile illness with constitutional symptoms and maculopapular/morbilliform rash	Bite of mosquito Vertical: usually *in utero*	Birds	Worldwide	Serology: antibody testing PCR
Yellow fever	Systemic: febrile illness with conjunctival injection; may progress to hepatitis or hemorrhagic fever	Bite of mosquito	Monkey	South America, Sub-Saharan Africa	
Zika	Systemic: febrile illness with constitutional symptoms, myalgia, arthralgia, retro-orbital pain, and scarlatiniform rash	Bite of mosquito Vertical: usually *in utero* Sexual contact Blood transfusion	Unclear	Central America, South America, Caribbean	

TREATMENT   Supportive

Explanation: This woman has Dengue. The classic signs and symptoms include high fever, retro-orbital pain, and an exanthem. Infections with this virus may present very similar to infections with Zika and Chikungunya which are also transmitted by mosquitos. Retro-orbital pain is more likely to be present in Dengue than in Zika and Chikungunya. Laboratory findings that are typical of infections with the Dengue virus include leukopenia, thrombocytopenia, and hypernatremia. There are four serotypes of Dengue. A person can be re-infected with any serotype more than once since the antibody response is not protective. Moreover, secondary infections are often more severe than the initial infection because of antibody-dependent enhancement. To date there is one vaccine available that targets all four serotypes of Dengue but it has not been approved for use in the United States.

Vignette: A 6-year-old boy in a rural village in Afghanistan presents to a clinic because he has been unable to use is left leg for the past week. The child's arm is weak as well. The boy has not received routine childhood vaccines. Fecal samples are sent to a large hospital in the nearest city and found to be positive for poliovirus.

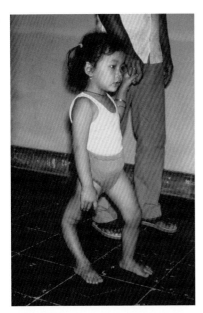

(1) *Source:* CDC public health library PHIL (phil.cdc.gov) image No. 5578
(http://phil.cdc.gov/phil/details_linked.asp?pid=5578)

8 Poliovirus

DESCRIPTION

Taxonomy: Picornavirus family.
See also ● 140, Non-polio Enterovirus ●; ● 89, Hepatitis A virus (HAV) ●; ● 33, Rhinovirus ●
Enterovirus genus (type C)
Virus properties: single-stranded, positive-sense RNA, non-enveloped

INFECTIONS
PRIMARY

Nervous: polio
    Subclinical (majority of cases)
    Minor illness
    Nonparalytic poliomyelitis
    Paralytic polio (1)

PATHOGENESIS

Paralytic polio: virus targets anterior horns of spinal cord and motor cortex of brain

EPIDEMIOLOGY

Transmission: fecal-oral
Polio is considered eradicated in most areas of the world.
Geographic distribution: to date, endemic in areas of Afghanistan, Pakistan, and Nigeria.

DIAGNOSIS

Serology: antibody testing
Viral culture

PREVENTION

Vaccination: inactivated vaccine and live attenuated (oral) vaccine

TREATMENT

Supportive

Explanation: As a result of effective vaccination efforts, polio has been eliminated from most countries. However, parts of Afghanistan, Pakistan, and Nigeria are still endemic. Major illness or paralytic polio is the least common form of polio but it is the most serious form of disease. This pathogen is part of the Picornavirus family, which includes enteroviruses such as coxsackie virus and rhinovirus and is transmitted via the fecal-oral route.

9 Rabies virus

Vignette: A 54-year-old man presents to a neurologist with weakness, pain, and tingling in his left arm and is diagnosed with neuropathy. A few weeks later, he presents to the emergency department with increased pain and weakness in his arm and with muscle twitching, difficulty swallowing and breathing, and increased salivation. The man is admitted and placed on ventilation. The man's wife recalls that about 1 month prior to the initial symptoms, a bat had flown into their bedroom and landed on the man's arm. Serology confirms the etiology. Two days after admission, the man becomes disoriented and combative. Four days following admission the man is in a coma. One week following admission, the patient dies.

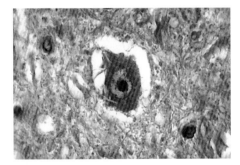

(1) *Source:* CDC/Dr. Daniel P. Perl
   CDC public health library PHIL (phil.cdc.gov) image No. 3408
   (http://phil.cdc.gov/phil/details_linked.asp?pid=3408)

9 Rabies virus

DESCRIPTION
Taxonomy: Rhabdovirus family; *Lyssavirus* genus
Virus properties: single-stranded, negative-sense RNA, enveloped

INFECTIONS
PRIMARY
Nervous:
Encephalitic/furious rabies: classic symptoms include hydrophobia, aerophobia, agitation and hyperactivity and eventually flaccid paralysis and coma
Paralytic rabies (rare): ascending paralysis—may mimic Guillain-Barré syndrome. *See also* ●62, *Campylobacter jejuni* ●

PATHOGENESIS
Virus enters via bite; virus G-protein binds to ACh receptor and neural cell adhesion molecule on host cell; virus replicates in muscles; enters peripheral nervous system; replicates in dorsal ganglia; travels in a retrograde manner to CNS; descends and disseminates via afferent neurons

EPIDEMIOLOGY
Zoonotic
Transmission: saliva/bite of rabid animal—common reservoirs include bats, small rodents, raccoons, skunks, dogs and cats

DIAGNOSIS
Microscopy: detection of Negri bodies (1), which are eosinophilic, cytoplasmic inclusions, in infected neurons
Serology: antibody testing
PCR

PREVENTION
Vaccine: live, attenuated vaccine
One of a few pathogens in which a vaccine can be administered after infection due to slow disease progression

TREATMENT
Treat wound; vaccinate; administer immunoglobulin; antiviral may or may not be utilized

Explanation: Rabies virus is a RNA virus that is transmitted via the bite of an animal. Common reservoirs include bats, small rodents, raccoons, skunks, dogs, and cats. The incubation phase may be several years, but is typically 1 to 2 months. Rabies begins with a prodrome phase that consists of nonspecific symptoms and then progresses to the neurologic symptoms as described in this case. Although the incubation phase may be long, the disease progresses rapidly once symptoms appear.

Micro gem: Alphaviruses are **ar**thropod **bo**rne viruses (**arbo**viruses)

Arbovirus is not a true taxonomic classification. Instead, it encompasses viruses from multiple families.

● 142, Rubella virus ● is also part of the Togavirus family, but is classified in a separate genus.

Vignette: A 63-year-old woman returns from a vacation to the Virgin Islands in the Caribbean. Her last 2 days there, she started feeling ill with a fever and just felt "bad." Three days after she returns from her trip she visits her primary care physician. She mentions she has had fever up to 39°C (102.2°F) and joint pain, and just yesterday she noticed a rash on her stomach. She also notifies the clinician that she received numerous mosquito bites while on vacation. At the time of her visit, her fever is 38.7°C (101.7°F) and a blanching maculopapular rash is observed on her trunk, back, and arms. The rest of her physical exam is normal. Serological testing demonstrates the presence of IgM antibody for a Chikungunya virus, which confirms the diagnosis.

DESCRIPTION

Taxonomy: Togavirus family; *Alphavirus* genus

Virus properties: single-stranded, positive-sense RNA, enveloped

Clinically significant viruses: Chikungunya, eastern equine encephalitis (EEE), western equine encephalitis (WEE), Venezuelan equine encephalitis (VEE)

INFECTION
 PRIMARY

Chikungunya

 Systemic: febrile illness with high fever, maculopapular rash, arthritis, and arthralgia

EEE, WEE, VEE

 Nervous: encephalitis

EPIDEMIOLOGY

Chikungunya

 Reservoir: primates

 Transmission:

  Bite of a mosquito (*Aedes aegypti* and *Aedes albopictus*)

   A. aegypti also transmits dengue, chikungunya, yellow fever, zika virus, and ● 7, Flavivirus ●

   A. albopictus also transmits dengue

  Vertical: usually perinatal

 Geographic distribution: endemic in West Africa; seen in Asia, Europe, Caribbean, North and South Americas

EEE, WEE, VEE

 Reservoir: birds, horses

 Transmission: bite of a mosquito

 Geographic distribution: depends on specific virus, North America, Central America, South America, Caribbean

DIAGNOSIS

Serology: antibody testing

PCR

TREATMENT

Supportive

Explanation: It may be difficult to distinguish Chikungunya from Dengue and Zika. All three viruses are transmitted by mosquitos and symptoms may be very similar and include fever, rash, headaches, arthralgia and myalgia. In this case, the serological analysis confirmed the identity of the causative agent.

Micro gem: *C. neoformans* is the most common agent of meningitis in individuals with AIDS

Vignette: A 40-year-old HIV-positive woman presents to the emergency department with a 1-week history of fever, malaise, and headache. Earlier that morning, her friend had stopped by to check on her and had found her confused and disoriented and had decided to bring her to the emergency department. On physical examination she is lethargic, her heart rate is 70 beats/min, her blood pressure is 100/60 mm Hg, and her temperature is 38.3°C (100.9°F). A head CT and lumbar puncture are performed. The head CT is normal, the CSF glucose is low, and the CSF protein is normal. Her CD4 T cell count is 87 cells/mm^3. No organisms are isolated from the CSF bacterial culture, but an India Ink stain is positive and encapsulated yeast cells are present.

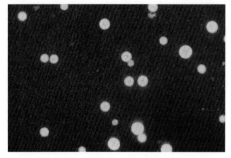

(1) *Source:* CDC
   CDC public health library PHIL (phil.cdc.gov) image No. 14391
   (http://phil.cdc.gov/phil/details_linked.asp?pid=14391)

11 *Cryptococcus neoformans* and *gatti*

DESCRIPTION Yeast

INFECTIONS

PRIMARY
Respiratory: pneumonia—primary focus of other infection types is lungs
Nervous: meningitis, meningoencephalitis

OTHER
Disseminated infections: may disseminate to any organ system
    Skin and soft tissue: lesions

PATHOGENESIS
Capsule
Melanin
Urease—breaks down urea and produces ammonia

EPIDEMIOLOGY
Natural inhabitant of the soil; enriched by pigeon droppings
Transmission: inhalation of yeast
C. neoformans
    Opportunistic pathogen
    High risk: immunocompromised, especially individuals with AIDS with CD4 T-cells < 100 cells/mm^3
C. gatti—may infect immunocompetent individuals

DIAGNOSIS
Microscopy:
    Histopathology—identification of yeast from pulmonary specimens
    Fontana-Masson stain will stain melanin
    India ink test positive (1)—encapsulated, budding yeast that do not uptake India ink

Serology: antigen testing by EIA, latex agglutination or lateral flow assay
Culture: Urease positive
    PUNCH = Urease positive organisms
        ●97, *Proteus mirabilis* ●; ●104, *Ureaplasma* ●; ●28, *Nocardia* ●; *Cryptococcus*; ●69, *Helicobacter* ●

TREATMENT
Depends on immune status and infection site—liposomal amphotericin B (may be used in conjunction with flucytosine), fluconazole

Explanation: The yeast *Cryptococcus neoformans* may cause meningitis and pulmonary infections, most often in the immunocompromised. This organism is equipped with a capsule and produces the enzyme urease to split urea. India Ink stain is the classic test for detection of this organism and demonstrates the presence of the budding encapsulated yeast. However, the India Ink test is not sensitive, hence antigen detection is currently the preferred method of diagnosis. Note that antigen based tests do not differentiate *Cryptococcus neoformans* from *Cryptococcus gattii*, a closely related pathogen. *C. gattii* causes similar infections but most often infects immunocompetent individuals and is more likely to cause mass lesions in the brain or lungs than *C. neoformans*.

Vignette: A 10-year-old girl is brought to the emergency department in July with a fever, headache, nausea, vomiting, and sensitivity to light of 3 days' duration. Her mother states the child recently returned from summer camp and had spent much of her time swimming in the lake. On examination her temperature is 38°C (100.4°F) and photophobia is observed. The CSF Gram stain is reported as "no organisms seen."

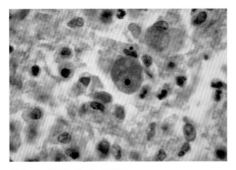

(1) *Source:* CDC/Dr. Martin D. Hicklin
   CDC public health library PHIL (phil.cdc.gov) image No. 323
   (http://phil.cdc.gov/phil/details_linked.asp?pid=323)

12 *Naegleria fowleri*

DESCRIPTION
Protozoa: amoeba
Free-living ameba—does not need human or animal host to complete its life cycle
Clinically significant morphological forms: cyst, trophozoite (1)

INFECTIONS
PRIMARY
Nervous: primary amebic meningoencephalitis (PAM)

PATHOGENESIS
Organism enters via the nose and travels to the nervous system via the cribriform plate

EPIDEMIOLOGY
Natural habitat is warm freshwater
Infections occur after contact with contaminated water following recreational activity, such as swimming, diving, and waterskiing
Transmission: inhalation of water containing cyst

DIAGNOSIS
Microscopy—identification of trophozoite from CSF
PCR available via CDC for confirmation

TREATMENT
High mortality due to rapid progression and difficulties in diagnosis
Amphotericin B may be used, but may not be curative
Miltefosine has shown activity against *N. fowleri*

Explanation: *Naegleria* is a parasite that is found in fresh water. The organism may cause primary amoebic meningoencephalitis. Although any age group is at risk for infections, children contract infections at a higher rate than other age groups. Transmission occurs via contact with contaminated water sources, and the pathogen gains entry into the nervous system via the cribriform plate.

13   *Taenia solium*

Micro gem: *Taenia solium* and ●87, *Taenia saginata* ● are closely related tapeworms. *T. saginata* or the beef tapeworm generally causes mild GI infections. In contrast, *T. solium*, the pork tapeworm may cause more serious infections, including neurocysticercosis.

Vignette: A 35-year-old man presents with seizures, headache, nausea, and vomiting. He had worked with the Peace Corps in El Salvador and returned to the United States about 8 months ago. Brain imaging demonstrates a cystic lesion in the cerebral cortex, with the presence of several scolices within the cavity.

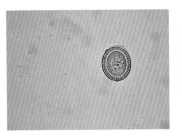

(1)

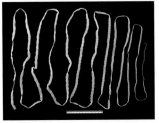

(2) *Source:* CDC public health library PHIL (phil.cdc.gov)
image No. 5260
(http://phil.cdc.gov/phil/details_linked.asp?pid=5260)

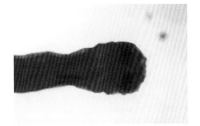

(3) *Source:* CDC/ Dr. Mae Melvin
CDC public health library PHIL
(phil.cdc.gov) image No. 10857
(http://phil.cdc.gov/phil/details
_linked.asp?pid=10857)

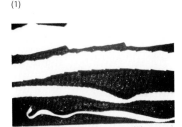

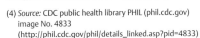

(4) *Source:* CDC public health library PHIL (phil.cdc.gov)
image No. 4833
(http://phil.cdc.gov/phil/details_linked.asp?pid=4833)

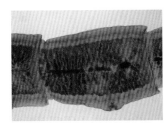

(5)

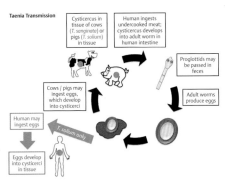

(6)

Taenia Transmission

- Cysticercus in tissue of cows (*T. saginata*) or pigs (*T. solium*) in tissue
- Human ingests undercooked meat; cysticercus develops into adult worm in human intestine
- Proglottids may be passed in feces
- Adult worms produce eggs
- Cows / pigs may ingest eggs, which develop into cysticerci
- Human may ingest eggs
- *T. solium* only
- Eggs develop into cysticerci in tissue

13 *Taenia solium*

DESCRIPTION

Platyhelminth / flatworm: cestode / tapeworm
Clinically significant morphological forms: ova (eggs) (1), adult worms (2), with scolex (head) (3), and proglottids (section of body) (4,5)
Alternative name: pork tapeworm

INFECTIONS

PRIMARY

Nervous: neurocysticercosis—lesions in brain due to larva in tissue
Note: larva may also disseminate to other tissue; brain is most common organ

OTHER

Gastrointestinal: tapeworm infestations—most often asymptomatic or mild GI symptoms

EPIDEMIOLOGY

Transmission (6)
    Tissue infection: ingestion of ova from food or water contaminated with human feces
    GI infection: ingestion of undercooked pork containing larvae
Geographic distribution: endemic in South America, Central America, Asia, sub-Saharan Africa

DIAGNOSIS

Tissue infection: most often diagnosed via clinical findings and imaging
GI infection: microscopy—identification of ova, proglottid or adult worm from stool
Serology: antibody testing

TREATMENT

Depends on infection site
Tissue infection: albendazole plus praziquantel
GI infection: praziquantel

Explanation: This is a case of neurocysticercosis caused by *Taenia solium*, a tapeworm. Human infections with *T. solium* can occur in two ways. In pigs, this pathogen is found in the larval form (cysticerci) embedded in muscles. Human ingestion of undercooked pork results in gastrointestinal infections due to cysticerci developing into adult worms in the small intestine. Adult worms lay eggs (ova) which may be passed into the stool of the infected individual. Ingestion of human fecal matter containing these eggs results in the formation of larvae (cystercerci) in human tissue, known as cysticercosis. One of the most common locations of dissemination is the nervous system. This organism is endemic in sub-Saharan Africa, India, and Central and South America. This pathogen should be included in the differential diagnosis of brain abscess, especially in immigrants from geographic areas in which infections are endemic.

14 Toxoplasma gondii

Micro gem: Toxoplasma and ●48, Cytomegalovirus (CMV)● are associated with AIDS-related retinitis.

Vignette: A 32-year-old, HIV-positive man presents to the emergency department with headache, fever, nausea, and vomiting. Earlier that day, his mother had stopped by to check on him because he had been sick all week. She decided to bring him to the emergency department because he failed to recognize her and because he seemed to be "talking nonsense." At the time of examination the man is disoriented, his temperature is 37.2°C (99°F), and his heart rate is 80 beats/min. His CD4 count is 60 cells/mm^3. The man has a history of infections with *Cryptosporidium* and *Pneumocystis*. A head CT scan reveals multiple ring-enhancing lesions in his brain.

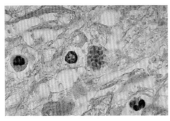

(1) *Source:* CDC/ Dr. Edwin P. Ewing, Jr.
CDC public health library PHIL (phil.cdc.gov)
image No. 575
(http://phil.cdc.gov/phil/details_linked.asp?pid=575)

Toxoplasma gondii: Transmission

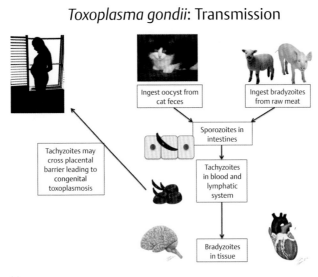

Ingest oocyst from cat feces

Ingest bradyzoites from raw meat

Sporozoites in intestines

Tachyzoites may cross placental barrier leading to congenital toxoplasmosis

Tachyzoites in blood and lymphatic system

Bradyzoites in tissue

(2)

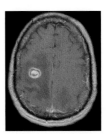

(3) *Source:* Thieme/Medlantis RadCases Case 074; Figure 4
(http://eradiology.thieme.com/?search=&q=toxoplasma&page=1&l=1&imageresults=on&videoresults=on&procedures=on&proceduresmedia=on&media=on&journalsmedia=on&pubmed=on&journals=on)

14 Toxoplasma gondii

DESCRIPTION
Protozoa: apicomplexia
Clinically significant morphological forms: oocyst (1)—several forms including bradyzoite and tachyzoite

INFECTIONS

PRIMARY
Immunocompetent are most often asymptomatic
Nervous: encephalitis, brain lesions
Congenital: mainly affects brain and eyes; chorioretinitis, hydrocephalus, intracranial calcification

OTHER
Respiratory: pneumonitis
Head and neck: eye—chorioretinitis

EPIDEMIOLOGY
Transmission (2):
   Post-natal: ingestion of cysts (commonly associated with undercooked meat or cat feces)
   Congenital—vertical (*in utero*)
   TORCH = congenital infections
   Toxoplasma gondii; **O**ther (● 106, *Treponema pallidum* ●; ● 117, Varicella-zoster virus ●; ● 55, Parvovirus B19 ●); ● 142, **R**ubella virus ●; ● 48, **C**ytomegalovirus (CMV) ●; ● 139, **H**erpes simplex virus (HSV)-1 and -2 ●
Opportunistic pathogen
High risk: immunocompromised, especially individuals with AIDS with CD4 T-cells < 100 cells/mm³

DIAGNOSIS
Serology: antibody testing
Microscopy—identification of trophozoites or cysts in tissue
PCR
Imaging studies may demonstrate ring-enhancing CNS lesions (3)

TREATMENT
Depends on immune status
Sulfadiazine, pyrimethamine

Explanation: *Toxoplasma gondii* is a parasite that can cause nervous system infections, especially CNS lesions, in the immunocompromised or congenital infections. The organism is transmitted via ingestion of the cyst in contaminated meat (most often pork or venison), ingestion of oocytes from contaminated cat feces, or vertical transmission from mother to fetus.

Micro gem: Two clinically significant branching gram-positive rods are *Actinomyces* and ●28, *Nocardia* ●. *Actinomyces* is anaerobic and not acid-fast and *Nocardia* is aerobic and is modified acid-fast.

Vignette: A 53-year-old man presents with a 1-week history of fever, facial swelling, and pain in his preauricular sinus and left cheek. Approximately 3 weeks prior to the symptoms, the patient underwent a tooth extraction. His temperature is 39.4°C (102.9°F). Physical examination reveals a small cyst on his left check, tender to the touch, and a discharging preauricular sinus. Gram stain of the discharge shows branching gram-positive rods.

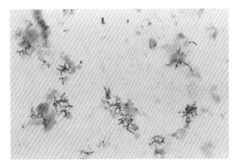

(1) *Source:* CDC/Dr. Lucille Georg
CDC public health library PHIL (phil.cdc.gov) image No. 10801
(http://phil.cdc.gov/phil/details_linked.asp?pid=10801)

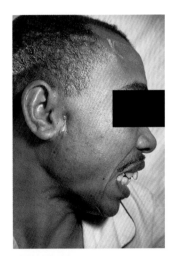

(2) *Source:* CDC/Dr. Thomas Sellers/Emory University
CDC public health library PHIL (phil.cdc.gov) image No. 2856
(http://phil.cdc.gov/phil/details_linked.asp?pid=2856)

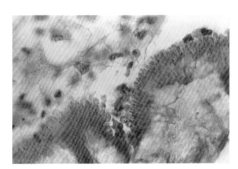

(3) *Source:* CDC/Dr. Lucille Georg
CDC public health library PHIL (phil.cdc.gov) image No. 14746
(http://phil.cdc.gov/phil/details_linked.asp?pid=14746)

15   *Actinomyces israelii*

DESCRIPTION

Gram-positive rods (1), branching, filamentous, beaded, thin
Facultative anaerobe
Many clinically significant species of *Actinomyces* including *A. israelii*

INFECTIONS
PRIMARY

Actinomycosis: chronic abscesses with draining sinus tracts
Head and neck (most common): cervicofacial actinomycosis—(2); often referred to as lumpy jaw

OTHER

Nervous: meningitis, meningoencephalitis, brain abscess, subdural empyema
Gastrointestinal: abdominal abscess
Respiratory: also called thoracic actinomycosis; pneumonia or abscess
Reproductive: pelvic abscess

EPIDEMIOLOGY

Normal microbiota of oral cavity, GI tract and female genital tract
Transmission: usually displacement of endogenous strains after breach in mucosa
Opportunistic pathogen
High risk:
  Cervicofacial actinomyces: poor dentition, dental manipulation
  Abdominal abscess: abdominal surgery or abdominal trauma
  Pelvic abscess: intrauterine devices

DIAGNOSIS

Microscopy: sinus tracts contain bright yellow pus with sulfur granules (*Actinomyces* filaments surrounded by PMNs (3))
Culture: slow-grower; on agar plate colonies resemble molar tooth

TREATMENT

Ampicillin, penicillin

Explanation: *Actinomyces israelii* is a branching, filamentous gram-positive rod. This organism may be normal microbiota of various areas of the body including the gingival crevices and tonsillar crypts of the oral cavity. Risk factors for oral infections include poor dentition and dental manipulation. Cervicofacial abscess may drain yellow exudate referred to as sulfur granules. It is important to differentiate this pathogen from *Nocardia*, which is also a branching gram-positive rod. *Actinomyces* is anaerobic while *Nocardia* is aerobic. Additionally, infections with *Actinomyces* produce sulfur granules while infections with *Nocardia* do not. Lastly, *Actinomyces* does not stain with the modified acid-fast stain while *Nocardia* is modified acid-fast.

Micro gem: Common bacterial agents of otitis media include *Moraxella catarrhalis*, ●136, *Streptococcus pneumoniae* ●, ●130, *Haemophilus influenzae* ●, and ●135, *Streptococcus pyogenes* ●
Common agents of AE-COPD include *M. catarrhalis*, *H. influenzae*, and *S. pneumoniae*

Vignette: A 67-year-old man with a history of COPD complains of worsening dyspnea and cough with increased sputum production. He has a history of smoking approximately 20 cigarettes per day for 20 years but has not smoked in 10 years. His temperature is 38.6°C (101.5°F), respiratory rate is 16 breaths/min, and forced expiratory volume in 1 second (FEV_1) is 75%. Course rhonchi and wheezing are heard on auscultation. After 2 days, his sputum grows gram-negative diplococci that are easily pushed across the agar surface.

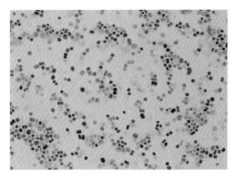

(1)

16 *Moraxella catarrhalis*

DESCRIPTION

Gram-negative diplococci (1)
See also ● 105, *Neisseria gonorrhoeae* ●; ● 4, *Neisseria meningitidis* ●

INFECTIONS

PRIMARY

Head and neck: ear—otitis media
Respiratory: acute exacerbation of COPD (AE-COPD)

EPIDEMIOLOGY

Normal upper respiratory microbiota
Transmission: displacement of endogenous strains

DIAGNOSIS

Culture

TREATMENT

Amoxicillin-clavulanate
Most strains produce beta-lactamases, which inactivate penicillins and cephalosporins

Explanation: This is an acute exacerbation of COPD. An acute exacerbation is a worsening of symptoms, especially a cough with increased sputum production. Exacerbations may be due to infectious agents, and the most common pathogens implicated include nontypeable *Haemophilus influenzae, Streptococcus pneumoniae,* and *Moraxella catarrhalis*. Of these, only *M. catarrhalis* is a gram-negative diplococcus. *M. catarrhalis* isolates are often described as hockey-puck–like, and they remain intact as they are pushed across the agar surface.

Micro gem: Both *Corynebacterium diphtheriae* and ● 133, *Pseudomonas aeruginosa* ● produce toxins that interact with EF-2 and inhibit protein synthesis. ● 71, *Shigella* ● and ● 65, Enterohemorrhagic *Escherichia coli* (EHEC) ● also produce toxins that inhibit protein synthesis, but by a different mechanism. These pathogens cleave the 28S RNA of 60S ribosome

Vignette: An 8-year-old girl wakes up with a sore throat and complains that she is extremely tired. She feels warm, so her mother takes her temperature, which is 38.9°C (102°F). Her mother notices that the girl's throat is slightly red. The next day, the patient stays home from school. On the third day, she still has the same symptoms and is having difficulties swallowing, so her mother takes her to the pediatrician. At the time of examination, the patient's temperature is 38.4°C (101.1°F). The physician notes a grayish-white exudate on the pharynx and severe cervical lymphadenopathy. The patient has not received routine childhood vaccinations

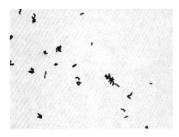

(1)

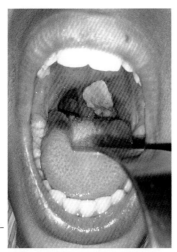

(2) *Source:* By User: Dileepunnikri (own work) [CC BY-SA 3.0 (http://creativecommons.org/licenses/by-sa/3.0)], via Wikimedia Commons (https://upload.wikimedia.org/wikipedia/commons/4/47/Dirty_white_pseudomembrane_classically_seen_in_diphtheria_2013-07-06_11-07.jpg)

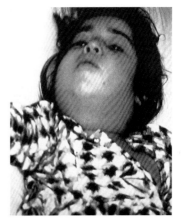

(3) *Source:* CDC
CDC public health library PHIL (phil.cdc.gov) image No. 5325
(http://phil.cdc.gov/phil/details_linked.asp?pid=5325)

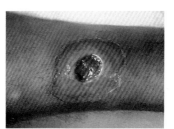

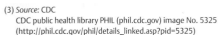

(4) *Source:* CDC
CDC public health library PHIL (phil.cdc.gov) image No. 1941
(http://phil.cdc.gov/phil/details_linked.asp?pid=1941)

DESCRIPTION   Gram-positive rods (1), club shaped, X- or Y-shaped, pleomorphic, palisading

INFECTIONS

PRIMARY   Diphtheria

Head and neck: pharynx—pharyngitis with pseudomembrane [grayish-white membrane composed (2) of dead cells, fibrin, RBCs, WBCs, and organisms]; severe cervical lymphadenopathy (bull's-neck appearance) (3)

Dissemination from respiratory tract may occur: myocarditis, neuropathy

OTHER   Skin/soft tissue: wounds/ulcer—cutaneous diphtheria (4)

PATHOGENESIS   Exotoxin/diphtheria toxin: ADP-ribosylates elongation factor-2 (EF-2) and inhibits protein synthesis; toxin is on a bacteriophage

EPIDEMIOLOGY   Transmission:

Pharyngeal diphtheria: respiratory droplets

Cutaneous diphtheria: contact with infected skin

High risk: unvaccinated individuals

DIAGNOSIS   Culture: grows on selective media such as Tellurite and Tinsdale

Definitive diagnosis: toxin detection

In the past the Elek (immunodiffusion) test was used; current toxin analysis is performed by PCR

Microscopy: detection of metachromatic granules, which are cytoplasmic granules in the cytoplasm of the bacterium that stain blueish-purple with methylene blue

PREVENTION   Vaccine: toxoid vaccines: DTaP, DT, Td, Tdap

TREATMENT   Antimicrobials (such as erythromycin) plus antitoxin

ANIMATION   http://go.thieme.com/microb/Video17.1

Explanation: *Corynebacterium diphtheriae* is a gram-positive rod (without spores) that causes diphtheria. The classic presentation of diphtheria includes the formation of a pseudomembrane, a grayish-white membrane that covers the pharynx that is composed of bacteria, debris, neutrophils, and fibrin. Another telltale sign of infection with this pathogen is severe cervical lymphadenopathy that gives individuals a "bull's-neck" appearance. This organism produces an exotoxin that inactivates elongation facter-2 (EF-2) and inhibits protein synthesis. Infections with this organism may be prevented with vaccination.

Micro gem: Adenovirus is a common agent of eye infections. Other important pathogens of the eye include ● 140, Non-polio enterovirus ●, ● 139, Herpes simplex virus (HSV)-1 and -2 ●, ● 100, *Chlamydia trachomatis* ●, ● 133, *Pseudomonas aeruginosa* ●, ● 136, *Streptococcus pneumoniae* ●, ● 130, *Haemophilus influenzae* ●, ● 134, *Staphylococcus aureus* ●, and ● 21, *Acanthamoeba* ●.

Vignette: A 12-year-old boy returns from summer camp complaining of a sore throat and red, itchy eyes. His mother takes him to the pediatrician's office where his temperature is 38.4°C (101.1°F). In addition, the physician notes that the boy's pharynx, tonsils, and eyes are red and inflamed, with the presence of cervical lymphadenopathy. The boy's mother states that he had been swimming frequently during camp, and that several of the other boys who also attended camp were experiencing similar symptoms.

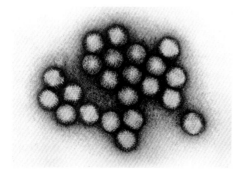

(1) *Source:* CDC/Dr. G William Gary, Jr.
    CDC public health library PHIL (phil.cdc.gov) image No. 10010
    (http://phil.cdc.gov/phil/details_linked.asp?pid=10010)

DESCRIPTION Virus properties: double-stranded DNA, non-enveloped (1)
Many serotypes due to fiber and base proteins—common serotypes are listed below with associated infections (not a complete list of all serotypes)

INFECTIONS
PRIMARY Head and neck:
Eye—pharyngoconjunctival fever (serotypes 3, 7), epidemic keratoconjunctivitis (serotypes 8, 19)
Ear—otitis media
Pharynx—pharyngitis
Respiratory: rhinitis, pneumonia, acute respiratory disease (ARD)

OTHER Gastrointestinal: enteritis (serotypes 40, 41)
Renal/urinary: hemorrhagic cystitis (serotypes 11, 21)

EPIDEMIOLOGY: Transmission:
Pharyngoconjunctival fever: respiratory droplets
GI: fecal-oral and fomites
Pharyngoconjunctival fever—associated with contaminated swimming pools
High risk:
Pharyngoconjunctival fever—infants and children
ARD-military recruits
Adenovirus is one of the most common agents of viral pharyngitis.

DIAGNOSIS Usually made on clinical manifestations
Viral culture
Serology: antibody testing
PCR

TREATMENT Reserved for severe cases and immunocompromised hosts
Cidofovir

Explanation: This boy most likely has a case of pharyngoconjunctival fever caused by adenovirus. Outbreaks of pharyngoconjunctival fever are associated with swimming in lakes or swimming pools. Adenovirus is a double-stranded DNA virus. It is one of the most common viral agents of pharyngitis. It also causes a variety of other respiratory infections, gastrointestinal infections, and genitourinary tract infections.

Vignette: An 11-year-old girl presents with swelling of the salivary glands. The mother states that her daughter is lethargic, complains of a headache, and has not been eating well for the past 3 days. The mother brought her daughter to the physician when she noticed swelling in her daughter's face. At the time of examination, the patient's temperature is 37.2°C (99.0°F) and severe parotitis is noted. She has not received routine childhood vaccinations.

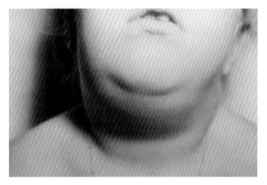

(1) *Source:* CDC/Dr. Herrmann
    CDC public health library PHIL (phil.cdc.gov) image No. 14488
    (http://phil.cdc.gov/phil/details_linked.asp?pid=14488)

19 Mumps virus

DESCRIPTION
Taxonomy: Paramyxovirus family; *Rubulavirus* genus
Virus properties: single-stranded, negative-sense RNA, enveloped
Only one serotype

INFECTIONS
Mumps

PRIMARY
Head and neck: parotid glands—parotitis (1) with fever

OTHER
Secondary sequelae
    Reproductive: oophoritis, orchitis that can result in male sterility/subfertility
    Head and neck: ear—hearing loss
    Nervous: meningitis

PATHOGENESIS
Initiates infection in upper respiratory tract and replicates locally then spreads via viremia to parotid gland and other organs.

EPIDEMIOLOGY
Transmission: respiratory droplets, fomites
High risk: unimmunized individuals

DIAGNOSIS
Serology: antibody testing
PCR
Viral culture

PREVENTION
Vaccination: measles–mumps–rubella (MMR), live-attenuated vaccine

TREATMENT
Supportive

Explanation: Mumps is part of the Paramyxovirus family (like ● 31, Parainfluenza virus ●, ● 32, Respiratory syncytial virus (RSV) ●, and ● 114, Measles virus ●) and is a single-stranded negative-sense RNA virus. The classic sign of mumps is parotitis or inflammation of the parotid glands. Complications of mumps include orchitis, oophoritis, and aseptic meningitis.

Vignette: A 54-year-old woman with uncontrolled diabetes presents with intermittent fever, facial pain, headache, double vision, and dizziness. She became concerned when a black lesion appeared on her nose. On examination, a nasal eschar is noted along with significant facial edema and periorbital edema. Her glucose is 780 mg/dL. CT shows thickening and bony destruction of the nasal sinus cavity and thickening of the medal rectus. Fungal stains from the eschar show broad, branching, aseptate hyphae.

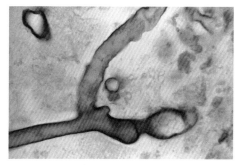

(1) *Source:* CDC/Dr. Lucille K. Georg
    CDC public health library PHIL (phil.cdc.gov) image No. 14551
    (http://phil.cdc.gov/phil/details_linked.asp?pid=14551)

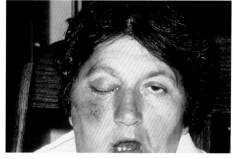

(2) *Source:* CDC/Dr. Lucille K. Georg
    CDC public health library PHIL (phil.cdc.gov) image No. 14810
    (http://phil.cdc.gov/phil/details_linked.asp?pid=14810)

20   *Mucor* and *Rhizopus*

DESCRIPTION
Important morphological form: hyphae—irregular, broad, wide-angled, branching, nonseptate or pauci septate (1)
Zygomycetes includes several genera including *Mucor* and *Rhizopus*

INFECTIONS
PRIMARY
Mucormycosis, also called zygomycosis
Head and neck, nervous: rhinocerebral zygomycosis (2)—starts as sinusitis that may progress to tissue necrosis with black eschar and destruction of turbinates

OTHER
Respiratory: pneumonia with necrosis
Skin/soft tissue: cellulitis that may develop into deeper abscess or ulcers
Gastrointestinal (rare): necrotic ulcers

PATHOGENESIS
Able to survive in high glucose and acidic conditions by production of ketone reductase

EPIDEMIOLOGY
Transmission:
    Inhalation of spores that may be in the environment
    Skin inoculation following trauma
Opportunistic pathogen
High-risk:
    Ketoacidotic diabetics
    Malnutrition/starvation
    Individuals with hematological malignancies
    Neutropenia

DIAGNOSIS
Fungal culture
Microscopy: identification of pauci-septate or non-septate ribbon-like wide-angled hyphae

TREATMENT
Liposomal amphotericin B, isuvuconazole

Explanation: Zygomycosis or mucormycosis may result in rhino-orbital-cerebral infections, as seen in this case. These infections most often affect diabetic patients in ketoacidosis. Zygomycetes are fungi and include several genera including *Mucor* and *Rhizopus*. These pathogens have the unique ability to survive in the high glucose and acidic conditions seen during ketoacidosis.

Vignette: A 24-year-old woman has been working long hours as part of her medical school surgery clerkship. Every day she comes home and falls asleep in her scrubs without removing her contacts. A few weeks later she is having difficulty seeing, and her left eye is painful and red, and the eyelid is swollen. Corneal scrapings are negative for bacterial pathogens, but fluorescent staining demonstrates the presence of trophozoites.

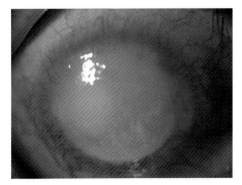

(1) By Jacob Lorenzo-Morales, Naveed A. Khan and Julia Walochnik [CC BY 2.0 (http://creativecommons.org/licenses/by/2.0)], via Wikimedia Commons (https://commons.wikimedia.org/wiki/File%3AParasite140120-fig1_Acanthamoeba_keratitis_Figure_1A.png)

DESCRIPTION
Protozoa: amoeba
Free-living ameba—does not need human or animal host to complete its life cycle
Clinically significant morphological forms: cyst, trophozoite

INFECTIONS
PRIMARY
Head and neck: eye—keratitis (1)

OTHER
Nervous: granulomatous amebic encephalitis

EPIDEMIOLOGY
Associated with soil and freshwater
Transmission
Keratitis: direct contact with eye
Encephalitis: inhalation, direct contact with skin following trauma
High risk for keratitis:
Poor contact lens hygiene, such as homemade saline solution, or cleaning contacts with tap water
Swimming while wearing contacts
Extended wear of contacts

DIAGNOSIS
Microscopy: identification of cyst and trophozoites from brain tissue or corneal scrapings

TREATMENT
Eye infections: chlorhexidine in combination with other agents

Explanation: *Acanthamoeba*, a parasite, may cause keratitis and is associated with extended contact lens wear, swimming and showering with contacts, or utilization of homemade saline solutions. This organism may also cause infections of the nervous system, especially encephalitis. The cyst and trophozoite forms of this organism may be recovered from tissue specimens.

Micro gem: *Onchocerca volvulus* is the second leading cause of infectious blindness worldwide. ● 100, *Chlamydia trachomatis* ● is the leading cause of infectious blindness.

Vignette: A 28-year-old man presents with a 3-week history of pruritus of his left forearm. His history is significant for recent travel to Ghana. A small pimple is observed on his arm. Skin snips demonstrate the presence of a filarial worm.

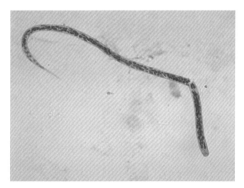

(1) *Source:* CDC/Dr. Lee Moore
CDC public health library PHIL (phil.cdc.gov) image No. 1147
(http://phil.cdc.gov/phil/details_linked.asp?pid=1147)

22 Onchocerca volvulus

DESCRIPTION
Nemathelminth / roundworm: filaria
Clinically significant morphological forms: microfilariae—larvae (1); filariae—adult worms

INFECTIONS
Head and neck: eye—river blindness
lesions, keratitis, uveitis

PRIMARY
Head and neck: eye—lesions, keratitis, uveitis
Skin: pruritic rash
Lymphatic: nodules in subcutaneous tissue

EPIDEMIOLOGY
Transmission: bite of a black fly
Geographic distribution: mainly in sub-Saharan Africa

DIAGNOSIS
Microscopy: identification of microfilaria from skin snip or other specimen
Serology: antibody and antigen testing
PCR
Evaluation of eye with slit lamp

TREATMENT
Ivermectin plus doxycycline

Explanation: Cutaneous infections with the nematode *Onchocerca* may manifest as nonspecific symptoms such as skin pruritus. This filarial worm may also cause more serious ocular infections, often referred to as river blindness.

Micro gem: *Bordetella pertussis* produces a toxin that interacts with G_i protein and increases cAMP. ●73, *Vibrio cholerae* ●, ●68, Enterotoxigenic *Escherichia coli* (ETEC) ●, ●61, *Bacillus cereus* ●, and ●109, *Bacillus anthracis* ● also produce toxins that increase cAMP, but these toxins interact with G_s protein.

Vignette: A 9-month-old girl presents to the emergency department with a cough. The mother states that the cough is repetitive and so severe that the child vomits after coughing. She also reports that the week prior, the child had a runny nose and seemed congested. The child has not received routine childhood vaccines. Upon examination, she seems ill and distressed. Her temperature is 37.7°C (99.9°F) and her lungs are clear. Numerous rapid coughs occur during the exam, which end with a long inhalation accompanied by a high-pitched sound, as well as cyanosis and vomiting.

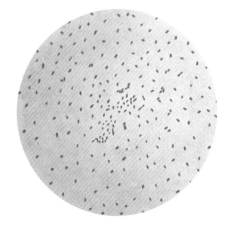

(1) *Source:* CDC
CDC public health library PHIL (phil.cdc.gov) image No. 2121
(http://phil.cdc.gov/phil/details_linked.asp?pid=2121)

DESCRIPTION   Short gram-negative rods or coccobacilli (1)

INFECTIONS
PRIMARY   Respiratory: pertussis (also called whooping cough)
Catarrhal stage: first 1–2 weeks—constitutional symptoms; highly infectious
Paroxysmal cough: lasts 2–8 weeks—paroxysmal cough with distinctive inspiratory whoop
Convalescence: lasts weeks to months—cough subsides

PATHOGENESIS   Exotoxin/pertussis toxin: ADP ribosylates G inhibitory protein (G_i) ultimately leading to increases in cAMP
Tracheal cytotoxin: destroys ciliated epithelial cells

EPIDEMIOLOGY   Transmission: respiratory droplets
High risk: unvaccinated individuals

DIAGNOSIS   Culture: grows on selective media such as Bordet-Gengou or Regan-Lowe agars
Serology: antibody testing
PCR
CBC: lymphocytosis may be present in infants and young children

PREVENTION   Vaccine: acellular vaccines—DTaP and Tdap
Vaccines do not confer lifelong immunity

TREATMENT   Azithromycin, clarithromycin

ANIMATION   http://go.thieme.com/microb/Video23.1

Explanation: This child most likely has pertussis caused by *Bordetella pertussis*, a gram-negative coccobacillus or short rod. This organism produces an exotoxin that increases cAMP. Pertussis occurs in three stages: (1) catarrhal stage—cold-like symptoms; (2) paroxysmal stage—classic paroxysmal cough with an inspiratory "whoop"; (3) convalescent stage—decrease in the severity of the cough and recovery.

Micro gem: *Chlamydophila pneumoniae,* ●27, *Mycoplasma pneumoniae* ●, and ●25, *Legionella pneumophila* ● are the most common bacterial agents of atypical pneumonia.

Vignette: A 68-year-old woman presents to her primary care physician with a cough of 2 weeks' duration, sinus pressure, and pain. She states that she had a sore throat one week ago. The cough at that time was nonproductive, but now she is producing a small amount of yellowish phlegm. At the time of the examination, her temperature is 37.8°C (100.0°F). Scattered rales in the left lower lung field are present. A chest X-ray reveals patchy areas of consolidation in the left lower lobe. Gram stain and culture of sputum are negative for organisms. *Chlamydophila pneumoniae* PCR is positive.

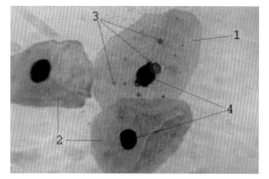

(1) Image by Eutensist, "Micrograph of *Chlamydophila* (*Chlamydia*) pneumoniae in an epithelial cell in acute bronchitis." Retrieved on May 9, 2016 from https://en.wikipedia.org/wiki/Chlamydophila_pneumoniae#/media/File:Chlamydia_pneumoniae.jpg.

DESCRIPTION
Rod-shaped
Cell wall has LPS but lacks peptidoglycan
Does not Gram stain
Cannot synthesize its own ATP
Morphological forms:
    Elementary body—infective, non-replicating form
    Reticulate body—noninfectious, replicating form

INFECTIONS
PRIMARY
Respiratory: bronchitis, atypical or "walking" pneumonia—most often community acquired
Infections with *C. psittaci* are commonly referred to as psittacosis or parrot fever

PATHOGENESIS
Obligate intracellular pathogens

EPIDEMIOLOGY
C. pneumoniae
    Transmission: respiratory secretions
    Association between *C. pneumoniae* infection and atherosclerosis
C. psittaci
    Associated with bird reservoir/exposure
    Transmission: inhalation of dried secretions from infected birds

DIAGNOSIS
Culture: does not grow in artificial media—use live cell culture
    In cell culture—large, cytoplasmic inclusions within epithelial cells will be seen (1); iodine may be used to better visualize inclusions
PCR
Serology: antigen testing

TREATMENT
Azithromycin, doxycycline

ANIMATION
http://go.thieme.com/microb/Video24.1

Explanation: This woman is most likely to have atypical pneumonia. Atypical pneumonia may be caused by several organisms, notably *Chlamydophila pneumoniae* and *psittaci*, *Mycoplasma pneumoniae*, and *Legionella pneumophilia*. *Legionella* most often affects older males so this is less likely to be the agent in this case. *C. psittaci* is associated with bird exposure and there is no indication of bird exposure in this case. This infection is most likely due to *C. pneumoniae* or *M. pneumoniae*. Neither *Chlamydophila* species nor *Mycoplasma* will Gram stain. Additionally, neither *Chlamydophila* or *Mycoplasma* grows on traditional media, such as blood agar and MacConkey. Most often a diagnosis is made by clinical findings. In this case PCR confirms diagnosis.

Vignette: A 67-year-old man presents to the emergency department with cough, fever, chills, and difficulty breathing. He reports that he is a hospital employee in the maintenance department, and last week he assisted with repairs to the hospital cooling system. He is a smoker and smokes one pack per day. His temperature at the time of examination is 39.8°C (103.6°F). His pulmonary examination demonstrates diffuse rales in the left lung field. A chest X-ray demonstrates diffuse patchy and interstitial opacities in the left lung. Sputum culture demonstrates the presence of gram-negative rods.

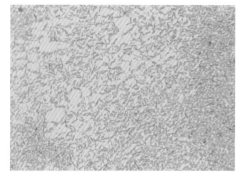

(1)

DESCRIPTION

Gram-negative rods (1)
Gram stains poorly because it is a very thin rod

INFECTIONS

PRIMARY

Respiratory: Legionnaire's disease—atypical or "walking" pneumonia that often progresses to consolidation; may be community-acquired pneumonia (CAP) or hospital-acquired pneumonia (HAP)

OTHER

Systemic: Pontiac fever—mild flu-like febrile disease

PATHOGENESIS

Facultative intracellular pathogen—replication in macrophages

EPIDEMIOLOGY

Normal inhabitant of water and soil
  Infections associated with water sources, such as cooling towers, whirlpool baths
Transmission: inhalation or aspiration of organism, most often from a water source; no person-to-person transmission
Typical patient is male, heavy smoker and drinker, > 50 years old, often with chronic lung disease
High risk: immunocompromised, especially individuals with cell-mediated deficiencies and transplant patients

DIAGNOSIS

Culture: grows on selective media—buffered charcoal yeast extract (BCYE) agar
Serology: antigen detection-urinary antigen test and direct immunofluorescence (DFA)
PCR

TREATMENT

Preferred: fluoroquinolones, such as levofloxacin, moxifloxacin;
Alternative: macrolides, such as azithromycin

ANIMATION

http://go.thieme.com/microb/Video25.1

Explanation: *Legionella pneumophila*, a gram-negative rod, may cause atypical pneumonia and is often associated with contaminated air-conditioning (cooling) or water systems often in large settings such as hospitals or hotels. It may also cause a milder, self-limiting, febrile disease, known as Pontiac fever. Smoking and underlying/chronic respiratory conditions increase the risk of infection with this organism. This organism can survive intracellularly by preventing phagolysosome fusion. Because this organism is intracellular, the host immune response is mainly cell mediated. Therefore, impaired cell-mediated immunity predisposes individuals to infections with this organism.

Vignette: A 50-year-old woman who has been incarcerated for the past 5 years is brought to the prison hospital with a cough productive of bloody sputum. She reports that the cough has been ongoing for approximately 2 months, but in the last few days she has noticed an increase in sputum production with the presence of blood. She claims she has lost approximately 20 pounds in the past few months and has had night sweats for about 1 month. She smokes 20 cigarettes per day, but the rest of her medical history is unremarkable. On examination she appears thin and frail. All her vital signs are normal. Her lung exam is notable for decreased breath sounds diffusely. A chest radiograph demonstrates a cavity infiltrate of the right upper lobe. A sputum specimen demonstrates the presence of acid-fast rods.

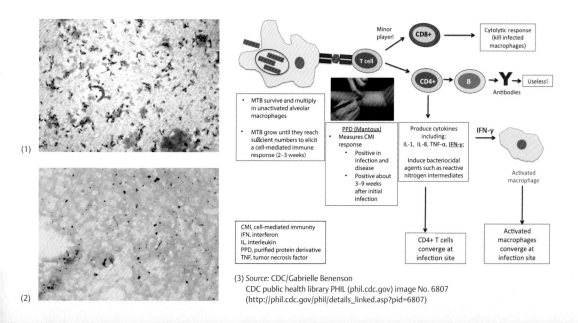

(1)

(2)

- MTB survive and multiply in unactivated alveolar macrophages
- MTB grow until they reach sufficient numbers to elicit a cell-mediated immune response (2–3 weeks)

CMI, cell-mediated immunity
IFN, interferon
IL, interleukin
PPD, purified protein derivative
TNF, tumor necrosis factor

PPD (Mantoux)
- Measures CMI response
  - Positive in infection and disease
  - Positive about 3–9 weeks after initial infection

Minor player!

CD8+ → Cytolytic response (kill infected macrophages)

T cell → CD4+ → B → Y → Useless!
Antibodies

Produce cytokines including:
IL-1, IL-8, TNF-α, IFN-γ;

Induce bacteriocidal agents such as reactive nitrogen intermediates

IFN-γ → Activated macrophage

CD4+ T cells converge at infection site

Activated macrophages converge at infection site

(3) *Source:* CDC/Gabrielle Benenson
CDC public health library PHIL (phil.cdc.gov) image No. 6807
(http://phil.cdc.gov/phil/details_linked.asp?pid=6807)

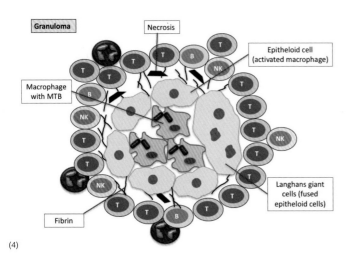

Granuloma

Necrosis

Epitheloid cell
(activated macrophage)

Macrophage
with MTB

Langhans giant
cells (fused
epitheloid cells)

Fibrin

(4)

DESCRIPTION

Acid-fast bacilli (AFB) (1,2)

Mycolic acid (a type of fatty acid) in cell wall

Does not Gram stain well: will see "ghost cells' or empty areas on Gram stain if AFB are present

MTB is part of the MTB complex, which includes *M. bovis, M. africanum,* and others

INFECTIONS

PRIMARY

Respiratory: pulmonary tuberculosis (TB)

Primary TB (infection): most often asymptomatic

MTB contained in granuloma (i.e., tuberculoma, Ghon complex) that eventually calcifies—granuloma typically in middle or lower lobe of lung

May remain latent indefinitely

Secondary TB (disease): classic symptoms include night sweats, weight loss, hemoptysis

Reactivation of primary TB

Granuloma liquefies releasing MTB, which can be coughed up or be released in the bloodstream resulting in miliary TB

Caseous cavitary lesion: usually in upper lobes of lung

May lead to extrapulmonary tuberculosis

OTHER

Extrapulmonary TB (also called miliary or disseminated TB): hematogenous spread of MTB; may disseminate to any organ system including:

Musculoskeletal: skeletal TB (Pott's disease), osteomyelitis

Nervous: meningitis, space-occupying lesions

Cardiovascular: pericarditis

Gastrointestinal: any location in GI tract or accessory organs including liver and pancreas

Adrenal: may lead to Addison's disease

Reproductive: prostatitis, salpingitis

Renal/urinary: renal TB or pyuria

PATHOGENESIS

MTB initially infects unactivated alveolar macrophages; survives and proliferates intracellularly (3); travels via lymphatics and disseminates to regional lymph nodes in lung; eventually macrophages are activated; macrophages and other immune cells migrate to infection site and granuloma forms (4)

Cord factor is produced in virulent strains

Causes "cording/roping of cells" microscopically

May inhibit PMNs

26 *Mycobacterium tuberculosis* (MTB)

EPIDEMIOLOGY

Transmission: person-to-person via droplet nuclei
Infectious during disease but not during latent period
Increased risk of transmission in close quarters, such as correctional facilities and homeless shelters
Immunosuppression, especially AIDS with CD4 T-cell < 200 cells/mm^3, increases risk of dissemination and reactivation

DIAGNOSIS

Screening test: Mantoux tuberculin skin test (purified protein derivative (PPD))
Positive test is induration > 5, 10, or 15 mm diameter (interpretation dependent on TB risk level of individual)
Note: measurement includes induration only and not erythema
Positive PPD test is an example of a type IV hypersensitivity reaction
Microscopy:
Acid-fast stains
Ziehl-Neelsen—"hot" stain (slides are heated while the primary stain is added)
Kinyoun—"cold" stain (heat is not necessary)
Acid-fast bacteria stain bright pink with Ziehl-Neelson and Kinyoun stains (1,2)
Auramine-rhodamine—fluorescent stain
Culture: slow-growing, selective media includes Lowenstein-Jensen, Middlebrook
Nucleic acid amplification
Immunodiagnostic tests to measure interferon-gamma (IFN-γ): quantiferon gold assay or TB Spot

PREVENTION

BCG (Bacillus Calmette-Guerin) vaccine protects against MTB. This vaccine is not routinely administered in the U.S. due to low infection rates. Individuals who receive this vaccine, such as immigrants, may subsequently develop false-positive PPD readings.

TREATMENT

Depends on several factors including immune status, infection or disease
Multidrug resistance is problematic
Effective agents include: **r**ifampin, **i**soniazid, **p**yrazinamide, and **e**thambutol (RIPE therapy)

Explanation: *Mycobacterium tuberculosis* is an acid-fast rod. One of the pathogenic features of this organism is the ability to survive within macrophages and prevent phagolysosome fusion. The classic presentation of tuberculosis includes hemoptysis, weight loss, night sweats, and the presence of a pulmonary cavity.

Vignette: A 24-year-old woman presents to her primary care physician with a cough of 2 weeks' duration and sinus pressure. She states that she had a sore throat a week ago, and the cough at that time was nonproductive, but now she is producing a small amount of sputum. At the time of examination her temperature is 37.8°C (100.0°F). Scattered rales in the left lower lung field are present. A chest X-ray reveals patchy infiltrates in the left lower lobe. The cold agglutinin titer is elevated.

DESCRIPTION

No cell wall
Does not Gram stain
Very tiny
Cell membrane contains sterols (cholesterol)

INFECTIONS

PRIMARY

Respiratory:
    Upper respiratory tract: pharyngitis, rhinitis, cough (non-productive or minimally productive)
    Lower respiratory tract: atypical or "walking" pneumonia—most often community-acquired

OTHER

Extrapulmonary secondary sequelae:
    Hematologic: hemolytic anemia
    Cardiovascular: myocarditis, pericarditis
    Musculoskeletal: arthralgias
    Skin and soft tissue: Stevens-Johnson syndrome (erythematous rash accompanies respiratory infections)

PATHOGENESIS

Induces inflammation
Induces production of IgM cold antibody

EPIDEMIOLOGY

Transmission: respiratory droplets
Pneumonia is most often community-acquired
High risk: school children and young adults in close quarters, such as military recruits and college students

DIAGNOSIS

Serology: antibody testing—IgM and IgG titers
    Cold agglutinin test for IgM—nonspecific for *M. pneumoniae*
Culture: requires serum for growth
PCR

TREATMENT

Doxycycline
Resistant to beta-lactam antibiotics due to lack of cell wall

Explanation: Atypical pneumonia may be caused by several organisms including *Mycoplasma pneumoniae*, ●24, *Chlamydophila (Chlamydia) pneumoniae* and *psittaci* ●, and ●25, *Legionella pneumophila* ●. *Mycoplasma* infections are often seen in children and young adults. Infections are referred to as walking pneumonia because often the patient seems well or better than what the chest X-ray indicates.

Vignette: A 53-year-old HIV-positive woman presents with fever, difficulty breathing, and a cough. On examination, her temperature is 38.4°C (101.1°F). The lung exam is unremarkable, but a chest X-ray demonstrates lobar consolidation of the left lung and pleural effusion. Gram stain of her sputum demonstrates branching, gram-positive rods that are modified acid fast.

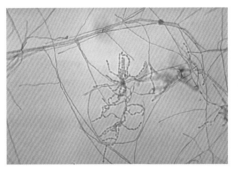

(1) *Source:* CDC/Dr. Lucille K. Georg
   CDC public health library PHIL (phil.cdc.gov) image No. 4232
   (http://phil.cdc.gov/phil/details_linked.asp?pid=4232)

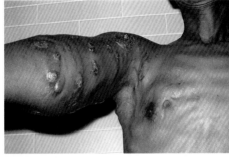

(2) *Source:* CDC/Dr. Libero Ajello
   CDC public health library PHIL (phil.cdc.gov) image No. 14749
   (http://phil.cdc.gov/phil/details_linked.asp?pid=14749)

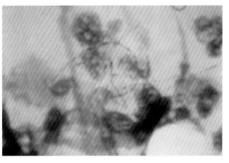

(3) *Source:* CDC/Dr. Hardin
   CDC public health library PHIL (phil.cdc.gov) image No. 15056
   (http://phil.cdc.gov/phil/details_linked.asp?pid=15056)

DESCRIPTION
Gram-positive rods, branching, filamentous, beaded (1)
Clinically significant species: *N. asteroides* complex (includes several species), *N. brasiliensis*

INFECTIONS

PRIMARY
Respiratory: pulmonary nocardiosis

OTHER
N. brasiliensis: Skin and soft tissue: abscess, cellulitis, mycetoma (2)
Disseminates to virtually any organ system
    Nervous : the brain is the common organ of dissemination; results in brain abscesses

EPIDEMIOLOGY
Found in soil/dirt and dust
Transmission:
    Pulmonary nocardiosis: inhalation from environment
    Skin and soft tissue: direct contact with contaminated soil, usually following trauma to the skin
    Ingestion (rare)
Opportunistic pathogen
High risk: individuals with decreased cell-mediated immunity
Dissemination is more likely in the immunocompromised

DIAGNOSIS
Culture—aerobic growth, urease positive
    PUNCH = urease positive organisms
    ● 97, **P**roteus mirabilis ●; ● 104, **U**reaplasma ●; **N**ocardia, ● 11, **C**ryptococcus neoformans and gatti ●; ● 69, **H**elicobacter pylori ●
Microscopic evaluation: partially acid-fast with modified acid-fast stain (3)

TREATMENT
Trimethoprim-sulfamethoxazole

Explanation: *Nocardia* is an aerobic, branching, gram-positive rod. This pathogen is an agent of respiratory infections and disseminated infections, especially of the nervous system and cutaneous infections. Immunocompromised patients are at higher risk for infections with this organism. Another organism to keep in mind when branching gram-positive bacilli are observed is ● 15, *Actinomyces* ●. *Actinomyces* is a facultative, anaerobic, gram-positive, branching bacillus that does not stain with the modified acid-fast stain. *Actinomyces* causes abscesses, especially cervicofacial, thoracic, abdominal and pelvic abscesses.

Vignette: A 25-year-old man who recently emigrated from Syria presents with fever, chills, cough, and shortness of breath. At examination, his temperature is 39.2°C (102.6°F), his respiratory rate is 28 breaths/min, and his oxygen saturation is 81%. Chest X-ray demonstrates the presence of bilateral infiltrates. PCR confirms the presence of a specific virus.

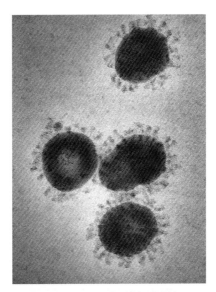

(1) *Source:* CDC/Dr. Fred Murphy; Sylvia Whitfield
    CDC public health library PHIL (phil.cdc.gov) image No. 15523
    (http://phil.cdc.gov/phil/details_linked.asp?pid=15523)

29 Coronavirus

DESCRIPTION

Taxonomy: Coronavirus family
Virus properties: single-stranded, positive-sense RNA; enveloped (1)
Clinically significant viruses: human coronaviruses (H-CoV), severe acute respiratory syndrome coronavirus (SARS-CoV), Middle East respiratory syndrome coronavirus (MERS-CoV)

INFECTIONS
PRIMARY

Respiratory
H-CoV: common cold (also called infectious rhinitis) and other upper respiratory infections
SARS-Co-V and MERS-Co-V: lower respiratory tract infections including pneumonia, acute respiratory distress
See also ● 33, Rhinovirus ●

EPIDEMIOLOGY

Transmission: respiratory droplets, fomites (important in transmission of common cold)
SARS and MERS: zoonotic—MERS associated with camels and bats
H-CoV: second most common agent of common cold (following rhinovirus)
Geographic distribution: MERS-CoV mainly seen in Middle East and northern Africa

DIAGNOSIS

H-CoV: diagnosis usually made from clinical findings
PCR
Serology: antigen testing- immunofluorescence
SARS-CoV and MERS-CoV
PCR
Serology: antibody testing

TREATMENT   Supportive

Explanation: MERS-CoV is a type of coronavirus that is most often seen in the Middle East and northern Africa. Although other coronaviruses are agents of mild upper respiratory tract infections, infections with MERS-CoV may be serious and locate to the lower respiratory tract resulting in pneumonia and respiratory distress. MERS-CoV can be diagnosed with PCR and serology.

Micro gem: Influenza viruses have a segmented genome.

Other clinically significant viruses with segmented genomes include ●6, Bunyaviruses●, such as California encephalitis virus, and Hantavirus and Reoviruses, such as ●49, Colorado tick virus ●.

Vignette: In January, a 62-year-old woman presents with a 3-day history of sore throat, runny nose, fever, and headache. She thought she had a cold, but she has also been experiencing chills and muscle aches, which prompted her to seek medical care. She has not been vaccinated for influenza this past year. Her temperature is 39.5°C (103.1°F), and the physical exam reveals pharyngeal erythema and mild cervical lymphadenopathy, but the pulmonary exam is unremarkable. A rapid influenza test is positive.

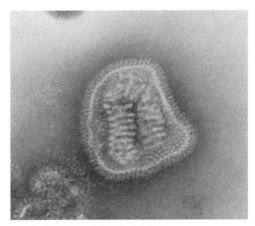

(1) *Source:* CDC/Erskine. L. Palmer, M.L. Martin
CDC public health library PHIL (phil.cdc.gov) image No. 8430
(http://phil.cdc.gov/phil/details_linked.asp?pid=8430)

30 Influenza virus

DESCRIPTION

Taxonomy: Orthomyxovirus family
Virus properties: single-stranded, negative-sense RNA, segmented genome, enveloped (1)
Important proteins:
HA (hemagglutinin): viral attachment protein
NA (neuroaminidase): cleaves sialic acid allowing release of newly made viral particle
M2: proton pump; acidifies vesicle during replication cycle
Clinically significant species: influenza A, B, and C viruses
Influenza A and B cause majority of infections

INFECTIONS
PRIMARY

Respiratory: flu—may manifest as common cold, sinusitis, pharyngitis, croup, bronchitis, bronchiolitis, or pneumonia
Secondary bacterial pneumonia may occur: most often with ●134, *Staphylococcus aureus*● or ●136, *Streptococcus pneumoniae*●

PATHOGENESIS

Antigenic variation
Antigenic drift: small gradual genetic changes (yearly vaccine changes); due to point mutations—contributes to epidemics
Antigenic shift: large and sudden genetic changes—due to reassortment of gene segments: contributes to pandemics

EPIDEMIOLOGY

Transmission: droplets or aerosols, fomites

DIAGNOSIS

Serology: antigen testing—rapid antigen assays using EIA or direct fluorescence antibody
Viral culture—cells infected with influenza virus will hemadsorb red blood cells to their outer membrane and cause agglutination of red blood cells due to viral hemagglutinin
PCR

PREVENTION

Vaccination recommended for all individuals > 6 months of age
Inactivated vaccine: intramuscular (IM)—quadrivalent or trivalent
Live attenuated vaccine ("FluMist"): quadrivalent
As of June 2016, not recommended
Recombinant influenza vaccine: IM—trivalent
Used for individuals with egg allergies

TREATMENT

For otherwise healthy patients, antivirals only indicated if administered within 48 hours of symptom onset
NA inhibitors: zanamivir, oseltamivir, peramivir
Note: amantadine and rimantadine that target M2 are no longer effective or recommended

Explanation: Influenza may be uncomplicated, as in this case, and is most often self-limiting. At times, more serious infections with this virus may also be observed and may include pneumonia caused by the virus itself or secondary bacterial pneumonia. Influenza is most common in the winter months, and infections may be prevented by yearly vaccinations. Due to antigenic variation of the virus, the vaccine must be reformulated yearly. Additionally, each influenza species contains several serotypes or subtypes based on envelope glycoproteins HA and NA. Influenza is a negative-stranded RNA virus.

Micro gem: Parainfluenza virus is the most common infectious agent of croup.

Vignette: A 3-year-old girl is brought to the emergency department by her mother with a 2-day history of cough and runny nose. The mother states the cough sounds harsh and barky, and there is a horrible sound when her daughter inhales. She also reports the cough is worse at night and causes her daughter to awaken. The patient's temperature is 38.4°C (101.1°F), and physical exam is unremarkable. She is up-to-date with all her routine childhood vaccines.

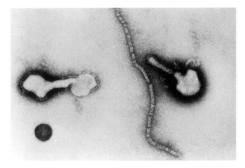

(1) *Source:* CDC/Dr. Erskine Palmer
   CDC public health library PHIL (phil.cdc.gov) image No. 271
   (http://phil.cdc.gov/phil/details_linked.asp?pid=271)

31 Parainfluenza virus

DESCRIPTION:

Taxonomy: Paramyxovirus family
See also ● 19, Mumps virus ●, ● 114, Measles virus ●, ● 32, Respiratory syncytial virus (RSV) ●
Virus properties: single-stranded, negative-sense RNA, enveloped (1)
Serotypes 1, 2, 3, and 4 are human pathogens

INFECTIONS
PRIMARY

Respiratory:
Young children: croup/laryngotracheobronchitis—classic symptom is "barking" or a "seal-like" cough—most often caused by serotypes 1 and 2
Children and immunocompromised adults: bronchitis, bronchiolitis, pneumonia
Immunocompetent adults: mild upper respiratory tract infections

EPIDEMIOLOGY

Transmission: respiratory droplets
Croup is mainly seen in young children ages 3–5 years old

DIAGNOSIS

Most often made clinically
Serology: antibody and antigen testing
Viral culture
PCR

TREATMENT

Supportive

Explanation: This child has croup. Croup is characterized by a seal-like, barky cough and is most often caused by parainfluenza virus. Parainfluenza virus is a single-stranded negative-sense RNA virus.

Micro gem: RSV is the most common cause of bronchiolitis in children <1 year old

Vignette: A 5-month-old boy presents in January with difficulty breathing. His mother states that he had a runny nose and mild cough about 3 days prior. At the time of examination, his temperature is 38.2°C (100.8°F), and tachypnea and mild expiratory wheezing are noted. Immunoassay demonstrates the presence of antigen to a specific virus.

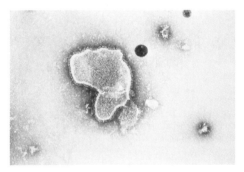

(1) *Source:* CDC/E.L. Palmer
   CDC public health library PHIL (phil.cdc.gov) image No. 2175
   (http://phil.cdc.gov/phil/details_linked.asp?pid=2175)

32 Respiratory syncytial virus (RSV)

DESCRIPTION

Taxonomy: Paramyxoviruses family; *Pneumovirus* genus
Two RSV subtypes (antigenic groups) mainly involved in infections: A and B
Subtype A causes more severe infections
Virus properties: single-stranded negative-sense RNA, enveloped (1)

INFECTIONS
PRIMARY

Respiratory
  Children < 1 year old: lower respiratory tract infections—bronchitis, bronchiolitis, croup, pneumonia
  Immunocompromised and elderly: lower respiratory tract infections
  Older children and adults: upper respiratory tract infections

EPIDEMIOLOGY

Transmission:
  Respiratory droplets
  Direct contact with secretions or infected individuals
  Fomites
Most often seen during winter months

DIAGNOSIS

Serology: antibody and antigen testing—rapid antigen assays
Viral culture
PCR

TREATMENT

Supportive
Ribavirin for severe cases

Explanation: This boy has an infection with respiratory syncytial virus (RSV). RSV may cause bronchiolitis, croup, or other respiratory tract infections. Infants and young children are at higher risk for infections with this virus than healthy adults. The incidence of infection is higher during the winter months. RSV is part of the Paramyxovirus family (like ●31, Parainfluenza virus ●, ●114, Measles virus ●, and ●19, Mumps viruses ●) and is a single-stranded, negative-sense RNA virus.

33 Rhinovirus

Micro gem: Most common infectious agent of the common cold (also called infectious rhinitis). Other common agents of the common cold are ●29, Coronavirus ●.

Vignette: A 31-year-old woman has a runny nose, stuffed sinuses, and sore throat, and she feels more tired than normal. A few days ago her husband came home from work with similar symptoms. She treats her symptoms with over-the-counter cold medications. After a week, the woman is back to her normal state of health.

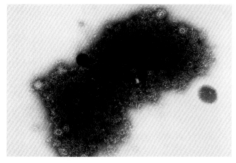

(1) *Source:* CDC/Dr. Erskine Palmer
CDC public health library PHIL (phil.cdc.gov) image No. 14618
(http://phil.cdc.gov/phil/details_linked.asp?pid=14618)

33 Rhinovirus

DESCRIPTION

Taxonomy: Picornavirus family
  See also ● 140, Non-polio Enterovirus ●; ● 8, Poliovirus ●;
  ● 89, Hepatitis A virus (HAV) ●
Virus properties: single-stranded positive-sense RNA, non-enveloped (1)

INFECTIONS
 PRIMARY

Respiratory: common cold (also called infectious rhinitis)

EPIDEMIOLOGY

Transmission: respiratory droplets, fomites
Many serotypes, which makes vaccine development difficult

DIAGNOSIS   Not usually performed

TREATMENT   Supportive

Explanation: There are many pathogens that may cause the common cold. The most common viral agents include Rhinovirus and human Coronavirus. These viruses are most often limited to the upper respiratory tract and cause mild, self-limiting infections, such as in this case.

34 *Aspergillus fumigatus*

Mico gem: *Aspergillus* hyphae branch at acute angles
Triple A: **A**spergillus—**A**cute—**A**ngles

Vignette: A 42-year-old woman with acute myeloid leukemia presents to the emergency department with a fever of 3 days' duration. She is currently undergoing chemotherapy for the leukemia. A CBC at the time of admission demonstrates a severe reduction in neutrophils. The woman states she has had a mild cough for several weeks, but, other than the fever, she has been feeling well. A chest radiograph demonstrates two cavities in the right upper lobe. A bronchoscopy with biopsy is performed and the bronchoalveolar lavage (BAL) fluid demonstrates branching, Y-shaped hyphae.

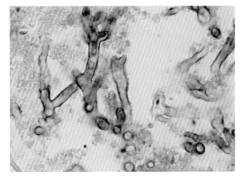

(1)

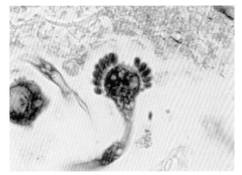

(2)

DESCRIPTION   Mold: hyphae are septate and branch at acute angles (1)

INFECTIONS

PRIMARY   Respiratory:
Allergic bronchopulmonary aspergillosis: associated with asthma and cystic fibrosis
Invasive infections: pulmonary aspergillosis
Chronic pulmonary aspergilloma (fungus ball)

OTHER   Dissemination from respiratory tract to:
Nervous system, cardiovascular system, skin and soft tissue, head and neck (rhinosinusitis)

EPIDEMIOLOGY   Transmission: inhalation of conidia (spores)
Opportunistic pathogen
High risk: individuals with neutropenia and impaired cell-mediated immunity

DIAGNOSIS   Fungal culture: microscopic identification of distinct conidia from colonies growing on culture plates (2)
Microscopy: identification of distinct branching hyphae from clinical specimens (1)
Serology: antibody and antigen testing
Aspergillus galactomannan antigen test—galactomannan is in cell wall of *Aspergillus*
Beta-D-glucan antigen—part of fungal cell wall; not specific for *Aspergillus*

TREATMENT   For invasive infections: voriconazole, isavuconazole

Explanation: *Aspergillus* is a fungus that may cause cutaneous infections, pulmonary infections, and disseminated extrapulmonary infections. The most common species involved in clinical infections are *A. fumigatus* and *A. flavus*. Invasive infections with *Aspergillus* are associated with immunocompromised individuals. The hyphae of this organism are quite distinct and are either Y-shaped or found as 45-degree angles.

Micro gem: *Blastomyces* yeast forms have a broad base
*B*lastomyces = **B**road **B**ase **B**udding yeast

Vignette: A 55-year-old woman who lives in Indiana presents to her primary care physician with cough, chills, fever, and difficulty breathing of 5 days' duration. She states that the cough began as nonproductive, and in the past few days has become productive of purulent sputum. A chest radiograph reveals alveolar infiltrates. Her bacterial sputum cultures are negative. A fungal smear demonstrates a broad-based budding yeast.

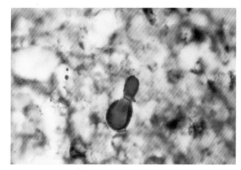

(1) *Source:* CDC/Dr. Libero Ajello
    CDC public health library PHIL (phil.cdc.gov) image No. 494
    (http://phil.cdc.gov/phil/details_linked.asp?pid=494)

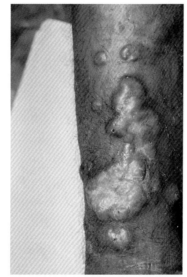

(2) *Source:* CDC/Dr. Lucille K. Georg
    CDC public health library PHIL (phil.cdc.gov) image No. 14877
    (http://phil.cdc.gov/phil/details_linked.asp?pid=14877)

35 *Blastomyces dermatitidis*

DESCRIPTION

Thermally dimorphic—exists as a mold at room temperature a yeast at body temperature
- 25°C: mold with pear-shaped conidia
- 37°C: budding yeast with broad base (1)

See also ● 37, *Histoplasma capsulatum* ●; ● 36, *Coccidioides immitis* and *posadasii* ●; ● 120, *Sporothrix schenckii* ●; ● 38, *Paracoccidioides brasiliensis* ●

INFECTIONS
PRIMARY

Most often asymptomatic
Respiratory: acute or chronic pneumonia, acute respiratory distress syndrome (ARDS)
Dissemination from respiratory tract to:
- Skin and soft tissue (2)
- Musculoskeletal system and bone
- Nervous system

EPIDEMIOLOGY

Associated with rotting wood
Transmission: inhalation of spores or contact with spores
Endemic fungus
- Geographic distribution: east of the Mississippi (MS) river (MS and Ohio River Valley)
Immunocompromised at increased risk for dissemination

DIAGNOSIS

Fungal culture
Microscopy: identification of budding yeast with broad base
Serology: antibody and antigen testing
PCR

TREATMENT

Liposomal amphotericin B

Explanation: *Blastomyces dermatitidis* is a dimorphic fungus that causes acute pneumonia, as in this case, or chronic respiratory infections. It may also cause extrapulmonary infections. This organism is endemic in the Ohio and Mississippi River valleys.

Micro gem: The endemic fungi include *Coccidioides*, *Blastomyces*, and *Histoplasma*.

Vignette: A 54-year-old man presents with fever, cough, muscle pain, chest pain, and night sweats. He states that he returned a few weeks ago from visiting his brother in Arizona and assisted his brother with building an addition to his house. His temperature is 39.8°C (103.6°F). Auscultation demonstrates the presence of rales and rhonchi. Several erythematous nodules are noted on his forearm. Chest X-ray shows patchy bilateral infiltrates. Serological testing confirms the diagnosis.

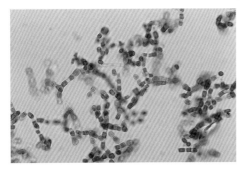 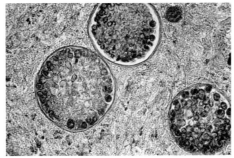

(1) *Source:* CDC/Dr. Lucille K. Georg
   CDC public health library PHIL (phil.cdc.gov) image No. 12196
   (http://phil.cdc.gov/phil/details_linked.asp?pid=12196)

(2) *Source:* CDC/Dr. Lucille K. Georg
   CDC public health library PHIL (phil.cdc.gov) image No. 14641
   (http://phil.cdc.gov/phil/details_linked.asp?pid=14461)

36 *Coccidioides immitis* and *posadasii*

DESCRIPTION

Thermally dimorphic—exists as a mold at room temperature a yeast at body temperature

25°C: mold with hyphae and arthroconidia (barrel or block shaped) (1)

37°C: round, thick-walled spherules filled with endospores (2)

NOTE: *Coccidioides* will not grow as a yeast in culture; spherules seen in tissue only

See also ● 37, *Histoplasma capsulatum* ●; ● 35, *Blastomyces dermatitidis* ●; ● 120, *Sporothrix schenckii* ●; ● 38, *Paracoccidioides brasiliensis* ●

INFECTIONS
PRIMARY

Most often asymptomatic

Respiratory: acute pneumonia, chronic pulmonary infections

Systemic: valley fever (respiratory and systemic manifestations)—subclinical /milder form of infection

Dissemination from respiratory tract to:

Nervous system, skin and soft tissue, and musculoskeletal system

EPIDEMIOLOGY

Transmission: inhalation of arthrospores from soil/dirt

Endemic fungus

Geographic distribution: Southwest U.S., Northern Mexico, *C. immitis*—San Joaquin Valley

Immunocompromised at increased risk for dissemination, especially individuals with AIDS with CD4 T-cells < 200 cells/mm³ (3)

DIAGNOSIS

Fungal culture

Microscopy: identification of thick-walled spherules from clinical specimens

Serology: antibody and antigen testing

Beta-D-glucan antigen—part of fungal cell wall; not specific for *C. immitis*

PCR

Skin test (not currently used): hypersensitivity to *Coccidioides* antigens

TREATMENT

Fluconazole, itraconazole

Explanation: This is an infection with *Coccidioides*. In the United States, *Coccidioides* infections are more common in western states such as California and Arizona. The pathogen is an inhabitant of soil, and infections occur after inhalation from contaminated dirt. Infections are often asymptomatic or subclinical. The primary site of infection is the respiratory tract, resulting in pneumonia and other pulmonary manifestations. Skin manifestations such as erythema nodosum, as in this case, may be observed in primary infections. In immunocompromised individuals, dissemination is common.

Vignette: A 54-year-old woman living in Michigan presents with a 4-day history of cough, fever, chills, muscle aches, and chest pain. She has been immunized for influenza and is up-to-date with all other immunizations. Her temperature at the time of the examination is 38.8°C (101.8°F). Auscultation reveals rales, and chest X-ray shows focal patchy infiltrates. Her rapid influenza test is negative. Beta-D-glucan is detected from her BAL, and an organism specific antigen test is positive.

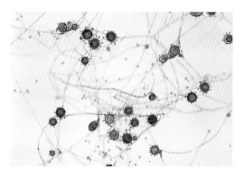

(1) *Source:* CDC/Dr. Libero Ajello
CDC public health library PHIL (phil.cdc.gov) image No. 10958
(http://phil.cdc.gov/phil/details_linked.asp?pid=10958)

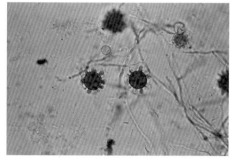

(2) *Source:* CDC/Dr. Libero Ajello
CDC public health library PHIL (phil.cdc.gov) image No. 15364
(http://phil.cdc.gov/phil/details_linked.asp?pid=15364)

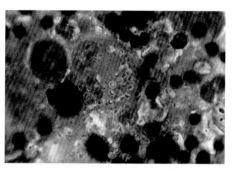

(2) *Source:* CDC/Dr. Lucille K. Georg
CDC public health library PHIL (phil.cdc.gov) image No. 1969
(http://phil.cdc.gov/phil/details_linked.asp?pid=1969)

37 *Histoplasma capsulatum*

DESCRIPTION
Thermally dimorphic—exists as a mold at room temperature a yeast at body temperature
- 25°C: mold with tuberculate (finger-like projections) macro-conidia (1,2)
- 37°C: budding yeast

See also ● 36, *Coccidioides immitis* and *posadasii* ●; ● 35, *Blastomyces dermatitidis* ●; ● 120, *Sporothrix schenckii* ●; ● 38, *Paracoccidioides brasiliensis* ●

INFECTIONS

PRIMARY
Most often asymptomatic
Respiratory: acute or chronic pneumonia, other pulmonary manifestations

OTHER
Dissemination from respiratory tract to:
- Adrenal glands, GI tract, nervous system, and skin and soft tissue

EPIDEMIOLOGY
Grows well in soil; growth enriched by bird or bat droppings
Transmission: inhalation of spores (microconidia) from soil
Endemic fungus
- Geographic distribution: east of the Mississippi (MS) river (MS and Ohio River Valley)
Immunocompromised at increased risk for dissemination, especially individuals with AIDS with CD4 T-cells < 100 cells/mm³ (3)

DIAGNOSIS
Fungal culture
Microscopy: identification of yeast in tissue; may be seen within reticuloendothelial cells/histocytes (3). *See also* ● 121, *Leishmania* ●; ● 103, *Klebsiella granulomatis* ●
Serology: *Histoplasma* antibody and antigen testing
- Beta-D-glucan antigen—part of fungal cell wall; not specific for *H. capsulatum*
PCR

TREATMENT
Pulmonary infections: liposomal amphotericin B followed by itraconazole,

Explanation: *Histoplasma capsulatum* is a dimorphic fungus that is endemic in the Mississippi and Ohio River valley area. This pathogen is transmitted via inhalation of pathogen that can be found in the soil. Soil enriched with bird or bat droppings enhances the growth of the pathogen. Most infections in immunocompetent individuals are asymptomatic. However, if symptoms are present, pulmonary manifestations as seen in this case are most common. In immunocompromised individuals, the pathogen disseminates to many organs, and symptoms vary based on the affected organ. There are several mechanisms of diagnosis, including antigen detection.

Vignette: A 64-year-old farmer in Brazil presents to the local clinic with a 3-week history of fever, cough, difficulty breathing, and weight loss. His temperature is 38.2°C (100.8°F). Lung exam reveals crackles, cervical lymphadenopathy, and pharyngeal lesions. Chest X-ray shows bilateral interstitial infiltrates. Large round yeast with several tiny daughter yeasts is seen on a KOH preparation from the sputum.

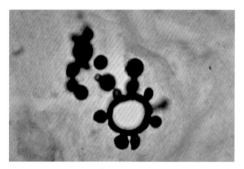

(1) *Source:* CDC/Dr. Lucille K. Georg
CDC public health library PHIL (phil.cdc.gov) image No. 527
(http://phil.cdc.gov/phil/details_linked.asp?pid=527)

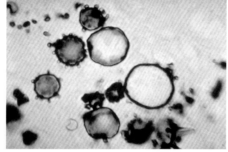

(2) *Source:* CDC/Dr. Lucille K. Georg
CDC public health library PHIL (phil.cdc.gov) image No. 520
(http://phil.cdc.gov/phil/details_linked.asp?pid=520)

38 *Paracoccidioides brasiliensis*

DESCRIPTION

Thermally dimorphic—exists as a mold at room temperature a yeast at body temperature
- 25°C: mold with septate hyphae
- 37°C: yeast—thick-walled mother yeast with multiple budding yeast; resembles "spokes of a wheel" or "pilot's or captain's wheel" (1,2)

See also ● 35, *Blastomyces dermatitidis* ●; ● 36, *Coccidioides immitis* and *posadasii* ●; ● 37, *Histoplasma capsulatum* ●; ● 120, *Sporothrix schenckii* ●

INFECTIONS

Primary infections are most often asymptomatic: granuloma forms at primary site; reactivation may lead to chronic infections

PRIMARY — Respiratory: pulmonary infection

OTHER — Lesions on mucous membranes and skin
Disseminated infection: many organ systems may be affected

PATHOGENESIS

Inhalation → Acute / subacute infection
↘ Granuloma → Latency → Reactivation → Chronic infection

EPIDEMIOLOGY

Transmission: inhalation of spores (conidia)
Geographic distribution: highest incidence in Central and South America
Immunocompromised at risk of greater disease severity and dissemination

DIAGNOSIS

Fungal culture
Microscopy: identification of wheel-shaped yeast from clinical specimens

TREATMENT

Depends on disease severity
Itraconazole, amphotericin B

Explanation: *Paracoccidioides brasiliensis* is a thermally dimorphic yeast that is mainly seen in Central and South America, especially in Brazil and surrounding countries. The yeast form is very distinct and resembles a wheel with a large central yeast and several daughter yeasts surrounding it. Infections arise following inhalation of pathogen. Once the pathogen is inhaled, a granuloma is formed at the primary site of infection, and following a period of latency, reactivation may occur, leading to chronic infections, which are most often observed in adults. Acute or subacute infections may also occur immediately following infection without latency. These infections are not common and mostly occur in children.

Vignette: A 54-year-old man, previously diagnosed with HIV, presents with fever, nonproductive cough, and difficulty breathing. His temperature at the time of the exam is 38.6°C (101.5°F), his respiratory rate is 30/min, and his O_2 saturation is 89%. Lung exam reveals course crackles throughout. His CD4 count is 74 cells/mm^3. The chest X-ray shows bilateral diffuse, finely granular interstitial infiltrates. A silver stain from the lung demonstrates the presence of cysts in the alveoli.

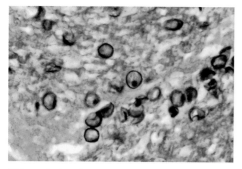

(1) *Source:* CDC/Dr. Edwin P. Ewing, Jr.
CDC public health library PHIL (phil.cdc.gov) image No. 960
(http://phil.cdc.gov/phil/details_linked.asp?pid=960)

DESCRIPTION

Previously classified as protozoan parasite
Clinically significant morphological forms: cyst—hat or disk shaped (1), trophozoite

INFECTIONS
PRIMARY

Primary infections are mostly asymptomatic
Respiratory: pneumonia
    Mainly associated with AIDS
    Also referred to as *Pneumocystis carinii* pneumonia (PCP)

EPIDEMIOLOGY

Transmission: inhalation
Opportunistic pathogen
High risk: individuals with defects in cell-mediated immunity, especially individuals with AIDS with CD4 T-cells < 200 cells/mm^3 and premature neonates

DIAGNOSIS

Microscopy: the Grocott's metheamine silver (GMS) stain is frequently used to identify *Pneumocystis*
PCR

PREVENTION

HIV-infected patients with CD4 T-cell count < 200 cells/mm^3 are recommended to take trimethoprim-sulfamethoxazole prophylactically to prevent PCP

TREATMENT

Trimethoprim-sulfamethoxazole

Explanation: This is a case of *Pneumocystis* pneumonia, and a typical chest X-ray shows diffuse, bilateral infiltrates. This pathogen is a fungus, but the morphological forms resemble protozoa and are referred to as trophozoites and cysts. Infections in healthy adults are most often asymptomatic but may be serious in individuals with AIDS.

Vignette: A previously healthy 61-year-old man presents with a 4-week history of a cough, productive of sputum. About 6 months prior, he had visited his family in Japan, and he recalls eating at an oceanfront seafood restaurant. He denies night sweats or any weight loss. His vitals and physical exam are unremarkable. CBC demonstrates eosinophilia. The AFB smear is negative. The sputum O&P exam demonstrates the presence of an ovum.

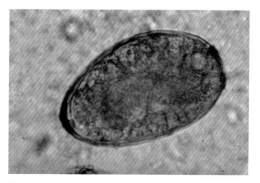

(1) *Source:* CDC public health library PHIL (phil.cdc.gov) image No. 4844
(http://phil.cdc.gov/phil/details_linked.asp?pid=4844)

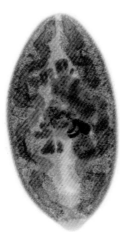

(2)

DESCRIPTION
Platyhelminth / flatworm: trematode / fluke
Clinically significant morphological forms: ova (eggs) (1), adults (2)
Alternative name: lung fluke

INFECTIONS
PRIMARY
Early infections—organism in GI tract then migrates to lungs
    Gastrointestinal: nonspecific/diarrhea
    Respiratory: cough, dyspnea, chest pain
Late infections—adult worm resides in lungs long-term
    Respiratory: inflammation and fibrosis of lungs; possible dissemination

LIFE CYCLE
Miracidia in snail: infects crustacean and develops into meta-cercaria; humans ingest crustacean; metacercaria excyst in upper GI tract and enter peritoneal cavity; migrate to the lungs and develops into adults; adults lays eggs; eggs are coughed up

EPIDEMIOLOGY
Transmission: ingestion of undercooked crabs or crayfish
Geographic distribution: mainly in Southeast Asia, but can be acquired in the U.S.

DIAGNOSIS
Microscopy: identification of ova from respiratory specimens (1)
Serology: antibody testing
CBC: eosinophilia may be present

TREATMENT
Praziquantel

Explanation: This man is infected with *Paragonimus westermani*, a fluke that is most often seen in East Asian countries, such as Japan. Early infections start with fever and GI symptoms. This is due to the presence of the pathogen in the GI tract. As the pathogen migrates to the lungs, pulmonary symptoms are noted. Infections may then progress to late infections, which mainly affect the lung. Late infections may closely resemble tuberculosis.

Micro gem: *Ehrlichia* and *Anaplasma* are transmitted by ticks
Other tick-borne pathogens include ●111, *Francisella tularensis* ● (tularensis), ●46, *Rickettsia* ●, ●125, *Borrelia burgdorferi* ● (Lyme disease), ●43, *Borrelia recurrentis* and *hermsii* ● (recurrent fever), and ●56, *Babesia microti* ●

Vignette: A 67-year-old woman presents with a 2-week history of generalized weakness, fever, and headache. She has a recent history of travel to Florida. At the time of the exam, her temperature is 38.7°C (101.7°F). Physical exam is unremarkable. Significant laboratory results are as follows:
CBC: WBC: 5.7 × 10⁹/L; platelets: 45 × 10⁹/L
Inclusions noted within monocytes
Liver function tests: AST: 679 U/L, ALT: 589 U/L

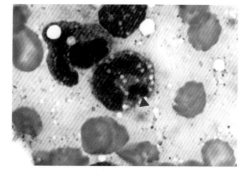

(1) *Source:* Safdar N, Love RB, Maki DG. March 2002. Severe Ehrlichia chaffeensis infection in a lung transplant recipient: a review of ehrlichiosis in the immunocompromised patient. Dispatch, Volume 8, Number 3.

41 *Ehrlichia* and *Anaplasma*

DESCRIPTION Gram-negative rods: Gram stain not routinely used to visualize
No LPS
No peptidoglycan
Clinically significant species: *E. chaffeensis, E. ewingii, A. phagocytophilum*

INFECTIONS Ehrlichiosis (also called human monocytic ehrlichiosis) and anaplasmosis (also called human monocytic anaplasmosis)

PRIMARY Systemic: febrile illness with nonspecific findings; rash may or may not be present

PATHOGENESIS Obligate intracellular pathogens
E. chaffeensis: infects monocytes
A. phagocytophilum: infects granulocytes

EPIDEMIOLOGY Transmission: tick bite (*Amblyomma*, which is also called lone star tick and *Ixodes*)
Geographic distribution
E. chaffeensis: Southeast U.S.
A. phagocytophilum: Northeast U.S.

DIAGNOSIS Blood smear: may show inclusion bodies termed morulae in cytoplasm of infected cell (1)
PCR
Serology: antibody testing

TREATMENT Doxycycline

Explanation: This woman most likely has an infection with *Ehrlichia*, an obligate intracellular pathogen. Inclusion bodies called morulae may be seen within the cytoplasm of monocytic cells. This infection is more likely to be caused by *Ehrlichia* rather than *Anaplasma*, because *Anaplasma* infects granulocytic cells and not monocytic cells. Infections are transmitted via a tick bite, and clinical manifestations may include fever, headache, arthralgias, and other nonspecific findings. Unlike another tick-borne infection, Rocky Mountain spotted fever (caused by *Rickettsia rickettsii*), ehrlichiosis and anaplasmosis rarely present with a rash. Laboratory results may aid in the diagnosis and may include leukopenia, thrombocytopenia, and elevated liver enzymes.

Vignette: An 8-year-old girl presents with a 1-week history of intermittent fever and loss of appetite. She has no significant medical history. She recently found a kitten on her doorstep that is now living with her family. The child's temperature is 38.4°F (101.1°F). She has scratch marks on her right arm, and her right axillary lymph nodes are swollen. Serology confirms *Bartonella henselae* as the causative agent.

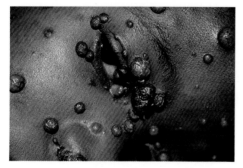

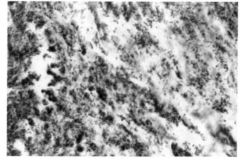

(1) *Source:* HIV.va.gov http://www.hiv.va.gov/provider/image-library/bartonella.asp?post=1&slide=352
George Beatty, MD, MPH, University of California San Francisco
Anna Lukusa, MD, Center for Infectious Disease Research, Lusaka, Zambia

(2) *Source:* https://en.wikipedia.org/wiki/Bartonella_henselae#/media/File:Blood_culture_negative_endocarditis.jpg
Photo: Warthin Starry, from traditional and molecular techniques for the study of emerging bacterial diseases: one laboratory's perspective. Emerg Infect Dis J 2002;8(2). CDC (http://www.cdc.gov/ncidod/eid/vol8no2/01-0141-G2.htm)

42　*Bartonella*

DESCRIPTION　Gram-negative rods or coccobacilli, pleomorphic
Clinically important species: *B. henselae, B. quintana, B. bacilliformis*

INFECTIONS
PRIMARY

B. henselae: cat-scratch disease
　　Lymphatic/systemic: febrile illness with regional lymphadenopathy
B. quintana:
　　Systemic: trench fever, also called quintan fever—recurring episodes of five days of fever followed by a five day afebrile period
B. henselae and B. quintana:
　　Skin and soft tissue: bacillary angiomatosis—vascular lesions that are most often on skin (1) but may also affect other organs
　　Cardiovascular: infective endocarditis—usually culture-negative
B. bacilliformis
　　Systemic: acute phase—Oroyo fever, also called Carrion's disease
　　Skin and soft tissue: verruga peruana-skin lesion—complication—hemolytic anemia

PATHOGENESIS　*B. bacilliformis* infects RBCs

EPIDEMIOLOGY　Transmission:
　　B. henselae: cat scratch or bite, flea bite
　　B. quintana: bite of louse (head, pubic or most often body lice)
　　B. bacilliformis: bite of sandfly
High-risk for bacillary angiomatosis: AIDS patients
Geographic distribution: *B. bacilliformis* infections mainly seen in South America

DIAGNOSIS　Culture: slow growers
Serology: antibody testing
Microscopy: Warthin-Starry silver stain for *B. henselae*—bacteria appear as black or dark clumps (2)
PCR

TREATMENT　Depends on species and immune status
Azithromycin, clindamycin, doxycycline

Explanation: *Bartonella* are gram-negative rods or coccobacilli. There are several species that infect humans, most commonly *B. henselae* and *B. quintana*. *B. henselae* often affects children and adolescents and is transmitted via the bite or scratch of a cat or a flea bite. Infections are referred to as cat-scratch disease and most often manifest as febrile illness with regional lymphadenopathy. Culture is not the best mechanism of diagnosis due to the slow growth of *Bartonella*; therefore, serology and PCR are preferred.

Micro gem: *Borrelia hermsii* is transmitted by lice.
Other lice-borne pathogens include ● 42, *Bartonella* ● (trench fever, bacillary angiomatosis) and ● 46, *Rickettsia* ●.

Vignette: A 37-year-old man in Ethiopia presents with a 3-day history of fever, chills, headache, myalgia, nausea, and vomiting. He reports that approximately 1 week ago he had experienced similar symptoms. His temperature is 38.9°C (102°F), and he is ill-appearing. Cardiac exam reveals a gallop. Other notable findings include hepatosplenomegaly. Blood smears demonstrate the presence of a spirochete.

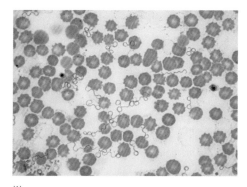

(1)

DESCRIPTION
Spirochete
Gram-negative cell wall—has an outer membrane and LPS
Does not Gram stain well

INFECTIONS
PRIMARY

Systemic: relapsing fever; repetitive cycles of abrupt onset of fever, lasting an average of 3 days followed by afebrile phase, which lasts about one week

PATHOGENESIS
Antigenic variation (pathogen changes antigen on cell surface), which leads to recurrent episodes of fever

EPIDEMIOLOGY
Transmission:
B. recurrentis: bite of a louse
B. hermsii and others: bite of a tick
Geographic distribution:
B. recurrentis: worldwide; endemic in parts of Africa
B. hermsii: worldwide; in U.S. mainly in West and Southwest

DIAGNOSIS
Microscopy: identification of spirochetes from Giemsa stained thick and thin smears (1)
PCR

TREATMENT
Penicillin
Jarisch-Herxheimer reaction may occur

Explanation: Relapsing fever can be transmitted by either lice or ticks. Louse-borne disease is endemic in select African countries. In relapsing fever, there is an abrupt onset of fever, chills, and other constitutional symptoms, which last a few days. During the afebrile period, the patient may feel well. After a few days or within 2 weeks, the fever and other symptoms occur again. Other findings of relapsing fever include hypotension, petechiae, and myocarditis.

44 *Brucella*

Micro gem: *Brucella,* ● 111, *Francisella tularensis* ●, and ● 127, *Coxiella burneti* ● are all zoonotic gram-negative coccobacilli that result in febrile disease. These pathogens are also agents of bioterrorism.

Vignette: A 51-year-old woman presents with a 1-week history of fever, chills, fatigue, and lower back and leg pain. She recently visited family members who live on a goat farm in rural India. Her temperature is 38.9°C (102.0°F). Physical exam reveals hepatosplenomegaly but is otherwise unremarkable. The complete blood count (CBC) demonstrates leukocytosis, and liver enzymes are elevated. Blood cultures are positive and demonstrate the presence of gram-negative coccobacilli.

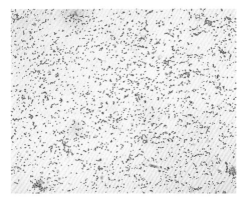

(1) *Source:* CDC/Larry Stauffer, Oregon State Public Health
Laboratory
CDC public health library PHIL (phil.cdc.gov) image No. 1901
(http://phil.cdc.gov/phil/details_linked.asp?pid=1901)

44 Brucella

DESCRIPTION

Gram-negative coccobacilli (1)
Clinically significant species include: *B. abortus*, *B. melitensis*, *B. suis*

INFECTIONS

Brucellosis: also called undulant fever, Bang's disease, and Malta fever
Infections may be acute or chronic

PRIMARY

Systemic: febrile illness that may affect any organ system; daily fever that peaks during late afternoon
Musculoskeletal: most common form that affects bones and joints

PATHOGENESIS

Facultative intracellular pathogen

EPIDEMIOLOGY

Zoonotic:
    B. abortus: associated with cattle
    B. melitensis: associated goats/sheep; most common clinically isolated species
    B. suis: associated with pigs
Transmission:
    Contact with infected animal
    Foodborne: commonly associated with unpasteurized milk, cheese
    Inhalation of contaminated dust

DIAGNOSIS

Culture: very slow-growing organism
    Appropriate safety precautions must be followed when working with this organism
Serology: antibody testing
PCR

TREATMENT

Doxycycline

Explanation: *Brucella* are zoonotic pathogens and are associated with a variety of animals including goats, cattle, sheep, and pigs. Infections are nonspecific; therefore, *Brucella* should be included in the differential diagnosis for a patient presenting with both fever of unknown origin and a history of exposure to the aforementioned animals. The most common manifestation is osteoarticular infections, which most often affect the sacroiliac joint and large joints of the lower limbs. *B. melitensis* is associated with goats, and infections most often arise after ingestion of unpasteurized milk or cheese or after direct contact with infected animals or contaminated secretions. This pathogen is a slow grower, and the clinical laboratory should be notified if this pathogen is suspected, as extreme precautions should be taken when working with clinical samples or with cultures.

Micro gem: Clinically significant spirochetes include *Leptospira interrogans,* ● 125, *Borrelia burgdorferi* ● (Lyme disease), ● 43, *Borrelia recurrentis and hermsii* ● (recurrent fever), and ● 106, *Treponema pallidum* ● (syphilis).

Vignette: A previously healthy 28-year-old man presents with fever, headache, and myalgia of 4 days' duration. He recently went canoeing on a river and at one point his canoe tipped over, and he was exposed to the water. He also recalls seeing rats along the bank. His temperature is 38.9°C (102.0°F). On physical exam, the patient's conjunctivae are red, but there is no discharge from either eye. Microscopic agglutination test (MAT) is elevated and confirms the identity of the causative agent.

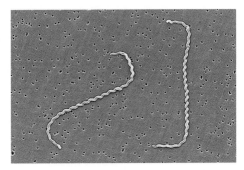

(1) *Source:* CDC/NCID/ Rob Weyant
    CDC public health library PHIL (phil.cdc.gov) image No. 1220
    (http://phil.cdc.gov/phil/details_linked.asp?pid=1220)

DESCRIPTION

Spirochete (1)
Gram-negative cell wall—has outer membrane and LPS
Does not Gram stain well

INFECTIONS

Leptospirosis: most often asymptomatic or mild self-limiting but if symptomatic, infections are biphasic with an acute phase and immune phase

PRIMARY

Acute phase
  Systemic: fever and other constitutional symptoms, conjunctival suffusion

OTHER

Immune phase
  Nervous: meningitis
  Renal/liver: Weil's disease—renal and hepatic dysfunction
  Respiratory: pulmonary hemorrhage syndrome

EPIDEMIOLOGY

Zoonotic: associated with many animals, especially rodents (especially rats), pigs, cows, horses
Transmission: contact with contaminated animal secretions (especially urine) or contact with contaminated soil containing animal secretions
Geographic distribution: more common in tropical climates; in the U.S., high incidence in Hawaii

DIAGNOSIS

During acute phase, pathogen is found in blood
During immune phase, pathogen is found in urine
Culture: slow grower; culture not routinely performed
PCR
Serology: microscopic agglutination test (MAT)—detects *Leptospira* antibodies from patient that agglutinate with known serotypes/antigens of *Leptospira*

TREATMENT

Penicillin, doxycycline
  Jarisch-Herxheimer reaction may occur

Explanation: This is a case of leptospirosis, a nonspecific febrile illness caused by the spirochete *Leptospira*. Although not always present, one of the distinguishing features of this infection is conjunctival suffusion, which is characterized by redness of the conjunctivae without discharge. Leptospirosis is typically associated with rats and infections are usually transmitted by contact with infected secretions, especially urine, from these animals or by contact with contaminated water. Infections are more common in tropical regions with heavy rainfall. In the United States there is an increased incidence of *Leptospira* in Hawaii. The microscopic agglutination test may be used to confirm the diagnosis.

Micro gem: *Rickettsia* are obligate intracellular bacteria, which means they must complete their life cycle and reproduce within the host cell. Other clinically significant obligate intracellular bacteria include ●100, *Chlamydia trachomatis* ● and ●41, *Ehrlichia* and *Anaplasma* ●.

Vignette: A 45-year-old man presents in August with a 3-day history of fever, headache, and muscle aches. He is an avid outdoorsman and recently returned from a rock climbing and hiking trip to the Smoky Mountains. His temperature is 40.1°C (104.2°F). An erythematous maculopapular rash is noted on his ankles and wrists. A CBC demonstrates a normal WBC count but decreased platelets. Serological testing confirms the diagnosis.

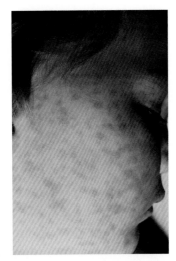

(1) *Source:* CDC public health library PHIL (phil.cdc.gov) image No. 14489
(http://phil.cdc.gov/phil/details_linked.asp?pid=14489)

46 *Rickettsia*

DESCRIPTION
Gram-negative coccobacillius
Very tiny
Does not Gram stain well
Cannot synthesize its own adenosine triphosphate (ATP)
Clinically significant species: *R. rickettsii, R. typhi, R. prowazekii, R. akari, Orientia tsutsugamushi*

INFECTIONS
PRIMARY   Systemic/skin and soft tissue: fever and rash

Organism	Disease	Signs and Symptoms	Vector
R. rickettsii	Rocky Mountain spotted fever (RMSF)	Constitutional symptoms Rash (1): maculopapular or petechial; starts at ankles/wrist and spreads to trunk; includes palms and soles	Tick
R. typhi	Murine (endemic typhus)	Constitutional symptoms Rash: maculopapular; starts at trunk and spreads; spares palms and soles	Flea
R. prowazekii	Epidemic typhus	Constitutional symptoms Rash: maculopapular; starts at trunk and spreads to extremities; spares palms and soles Brill-Zinsser disease- recurrence of infection years after initial episode; milder disease	Louse
R. akari	Rickettsialpox	Lesion: papule that develops into vesicle then eschar that crusts Constitutional symptoms Rash: generalized papular or vesicular rash	Mite
O. tsutsugamushi	Scrub typhus	Lesion at bite site: papule that develops into ulcer; then eschar that crusts Constitutional symptoms Rash: macular starts on trunk and spreads to extremities; lymphadenopathy	Mite

PATHOGENESIS   Obligate intracellular pathogens

EPIDEMIOLOGY   Transmission: bite of arthropod vector
Geographical distribution: most seen worldwide; *O. tsutsugamushi* mainly in East Asia

DIAGNOSIS   Does not grow on routine microbiological media: will grow in cell culture
Serology: antibody testing for definitive diagnosis
  In the past, Weil-Felix test was used but this test is no longer used

TREATMENT   Doxycycline

Explanation: Rocky Mountain spotted fever (RMSF) is caused by *Rickettsia rickettsii*. *R. rickettsii* is the most commonly seen species of *Rickettsia* seen in the United States. Infections are transmitted by several species of ticks, including the American dog tick (*Dermacentor variabilis*), the Rocky Mountain wood tick (*Dermacentor andersoni*), and the brown dog tick (*Rhipicephalus sanguineus*). Classic symptoms include constitutional symptoms, such as seen in this case, and a rash that starts on the extremities and eventually spreads inward to the trunk. This pathogen preferentially infects vascular endothelial cells, which may result in thrombocytopenia. Another rickettsial pathogen, *R. prowazekii*, is the agent of epidemic typhus, and the symptoms are very similar to RMSF. However, the rash of epidemic typhus starts on the trunk and spreads to the extremities.

Vignette: A 22-year-old female college student presented to the university clinic with fever, chills, and headache of 1-week duration. Prior to the onset of the fever and chills, she experienced abdominal pain and mild diarrhea. She recently returned from a semester abroad in India. She had refused all travel vaccinations prior to her trip. Her temperature is 39.1°C (102.4°F). Lymphadenopathy is not observed on examination. Her abdomen is tender, and there is no liver or spleen enlargement. Thick and thin films for ● 59, *Plasmodium* ● are negative. After 2 days, blood cultures grow gram-negative rods that are lactose negative on MacConkey agar.

(1)

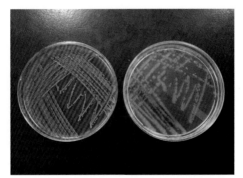

(2) *Source:* CDC/Armed Forces Institute of Pathology, Charles N. Farmer
CDC public health library PHIL (phil.cdc.gov) image No. 2215
(http://phil.cdc.gov/phil/details_linked.asp?pid=2215)

(3) MacConkey agar. Left, lactose positive. Right, lactose negative.

DESCRIPTION

Gram-negative rods (1); part of *Enterobacteriaceae* family
See also ●129, *Escherichia coli* ●; ●103, *Klebsiella granulomatis* ●; ●113, *Klebsiella pneumoniae* ●; ●97, *Proteus* ●; ●70, Nontyphoidal *Salmonella* ●; ●71, *Shigella* ●; ●74, *Yersinia enterocolitica* and *pseudotuberculosis* ●; ●138, *Yersinia pestis* ●

INFECTIONS
PRIMARY

Systemic: typhoid/enteric fever—fever, chills, abdominal pain, maculopapular rash (called rose spots) (2), hepatosplenomegaly
     Complication—intestinal bleeding

PATHOGENESIS

LPS
Capsule (Vi antigen)
Invasion of cells and intracellular survival

EPIDEMIOLOGY

Solely a human pathogen
Transmission: fecal-oral
Organism can colonize gallbladder, leading to a chronic carrier state
Asymptomatic carriers are infectious
Endemic in areas of overcrowding and poor sanitation

DIAGNOSIS

Culture: lactose negative (3), *S. typhi* is H_2S positive
Serology: Widal test—detects antibodies from the patient using known antigens to *S. typhi* or *paratyphi*

PREVENTION

Typhoid vaccines:
     Ty21a—live vaccine; oral administration
     Vi—polysaccharide vaccine, parenteral administration

TREATMENT

Ciprofloxacin, levofloxacin, ceftriaxone

ANIMATION

http://go.thieme.com/microb/Video47.1

Explanation: This woman has an infection with *Salmonella enterica* serotype typhi, a lactose-negative, gram-negative rod that causes the febrile illness, typhoid fever. MacConkey agar will only grow gram-negative bacteria and lactose fermenting colonies will appear pink, whereas non-lactose fermenting colonies will be colorless. Travelers to endemic regions are at high risk for infections, and vaccination prior to travel is recommended. It is important to note that the typhoid vaccines do not provide absolute protection from *S. typhi* or from *S. paratyphi*, which may also cause typhoid fever.

Micro gem: The three main pathogens associated with AIDS-related esophagitis (in order of frequency) are ●143, *Candida* species ●, Cytomegalovirus, and ●139, Herpes simplex virus (HSV)-1 and -2 ●.

Vignette: A 47-year-old HIV-positive woman presents with a several-week history of weight loss, abdominal pain, and watery diarrhea. She reports that she frequently needs to empty her bowels, and she noticed blood in her stools recently. She has lost 15 pounds in the last few weeks. She has previously been diagnosed with HIV but is not currently receiving care or taking medication for the HIV infection. Her CD4 count is 38 cells/mm^3. A colonoscopy shows inflammation of the colonic mucosa and the presence of ulcers and erosions. A biopsy is sent for histological staining, and it shows enlarged cells with eccentric, basophilic intranuclear inclusions.

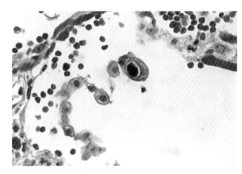

(1) *Source:* CDC/Dr. Edwin P. Ewing, Jr.
   CDC public health library PHIL (phil.cdc.gov) image No. 958
   (http://phil.cdc.gov/phil/details_linked.asp?pid=958)

48 Cytomegalovirus (CMV)

DESCRIPTION

Taxonomy: Herpesvirus family
See also ●51, Epstein-Barr virus (EBV)●; ●139, Herpes simplex virus (HSV)-1 and -2 ●; ●52, Human herpes virus-6 (HHV-6)●; ●117, Varicella-zoster virus ●
Virus properties: double-stranded DNA, enveloped
Also called human herpes virus-5

INFECTIONS
PRIMARY

Mainly asymptomatic in immunocompetent host
Immunocompetent host
    Systemic: infectious mononucleosis
        See also ●51, Epstein-Barr virus (EBV) ●
AIDS related
    Gastrointestinal: esophagitis, colitis
        See also ●139, Herpes simplex virus (HSV)-1 and -2 ●;
        ●143, *Candida* species ●
    Head and Neck: eye—retinitis
        See also ●14, *Toxoplasma gondii* ●
    Respiratory: pneumonia
Congenital
    Cardiovascular: patent ductus arteriosus and pulmonary artery hypoplasia
    Head and neck: ear—hearing loss; eye: cataracts
    Nervous: seizures and other neurologic issues
    Skin and soft tissue: petechiae ("blueberry muffin" rash)
    TORCH = congenital infections
    ●14, **T**oxoplasma gondii ●; **O**ther (●106, *Treponema pallidum* ●; ●117, Varicella-zoster virus ●; ●55, Parvovirus B19 ●); ●142, **R**ubella virus ●; **C**ytomegalovirus; ●139, **H**erpes simplex virus (HSV)-1 and -2 ●

PATHOGENESIS

Infects epithelial cells, lymphocytes, and other cells
Remains latent in monocytic cells and other cells

EPIDEMIOLOGY

Transmission:
    Direct contact with saliva, urine, breast milk
    Sexual contact
    Vertical: most often *in utero*
    Blood transfusion
    Organ transplant
Opportunistic pathogen
High risk: immunocompromised, especially individuals with AIDS with CD4 T-cells < 50 cells/mm^3 and transplant recipients

DIAGNOSIS

Viral culture
Microscopy: identification of large cells with inclusion bodies ("owl-eye" inclusions) (1)
Serology: antigen and antibody detection
    CMV infectious mononucleosis = heterophile antibody negative
PCR

TREATMENT

Immunocompetent: no treatment recommended
Valganciclovir, ganciclovir

Explanation: This is an infection with CMV. CMV is frequently associated with AIDS and commonly affects the GI tract, lungs, or eyes. Although any part of the GI tract may be infected, the esophagus and colon are most often involved. Clinical manifestations of CMV colitis may include weight loss, abdominal pain, diarrhea, and low-grade fever. Tenesmus and hematochezia may be present as well. One mechanism of identifying CMV is histological staining of biopsy specimens from the colon. Cytomegalic cells with intranuclear inclusions may be observed. These inclusions are often referred to as owl-eye inclusions.

Vignette: A 20-year-old college student returns from a Rocky Mountain summer hiking trip feeling sick. For 2 days he stays home from his summer job mowing lawns, and on the third day he feels better and returns to work. After 3 days his fever returns, and at the urging of his mother, he goes to the emergency department. In addition to the fever, he complains of headache, muscle ache, and fatigue. He reports that while camping in the Rockies his girlfriend had removed a tick from his back. His temperature is 39.4°C (102.9°F). His physical exam is unremarkable. Serological testing for *Rickettsia, Ehrlichia* and *Anaplasma, Borrelia recurrentis* and *hermsii,* and *Francisella tularensis* is negative. Thick and thin smears are negative for *Babesia*. An additional serological test is positive and confirms the diagnosis.

49 Colorado tick virus

DESCRIPTION

Taxonomy: Reovirus family; *Coltivirus* genus
Virus properties: double-stranded DNA, segmented genome, non-enveloped
Arbovirus—Arbovirus is not a true taxonomic classification.
  See also ●10, Alphavirus ●, ●7, Arthopod borne Flavivirus ●, and ●6, Bunyavirus ●
Instead, it encompasses viruses from multiple families.
  See also ●76, Rotavirus ●

INFECTIONS
PRIMARY

Colorado tick fever
Systemic: biphasic fever with petechial or maculopapular rash

EPIDEMIOLOGY

Transmission: bite of tick (vector)
Reservoir: rodents
Geographic distribution: Western U.S.

PATHOGENENSIS   Infects RBCs

DIAGNOSIS   Serology: antibody testing
PCR

TREATMENT   Supportive

Explanation: This man has Colorado tick fever. This infection is mainly seen in the western part of the United States in the summer months and is transmitted by the bite of a tick. A key characteristic of this infection is the biphasic nature of the fever. Individuals are febrile for 2 to 3 days followed by a 2- to 3-day afebrile period. It is important to distinguish this pathogen from other infections that are also tick borne. Serological tests are available for many of the tick-borne diseases, including Colorado tick fever.

Vignette: A 45-year-old woman presents with fever of up to 38.9°C (102.0°F), malaise, and headache. She states the symptoms started suddenly 2 days ago, and she is now also experiencing diarrhea, nausea, and vomiting. Two weeks ago she returned from a medical mission trip to the Democratic Republic of Congo. Her temperature at the time of the exam is 39.3°C (102.7°F). Pharyngitis and conjunctivitis are noted on physical exam. Laboratory analysis reveals decreased WBCs, decreased platelets, and elevated liver function tests. She is placed in isolation as a precaution, and a blood sample is sent to the CDC for analysis. Reverse-transcriptase polymerase chain reaction (RT-PCR) confirms the identity of the pathogenic agent of this infection.

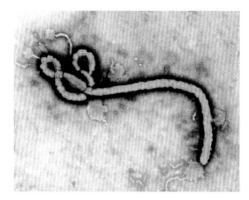

(1) *Source:* CDC public health library PHIL (phil.cdc.gov) image
No. 10815
(http://phil.cdc.gov/phil/details_linked.asp?pid=10815)

DESCRIPTION

Taxonomy: Filovirus family

Virus properties: single-stranded, negative-sense RNA, enveloped (1)

INFECTIONS
PRIMARY

Ebola and Marburg virus infections

Systemic: febrile illness with maculopapular rash; hemorrhagic form of infection may occur

EPIDEMIOLOGY

Zoonotic

Transmission:

    Contact with infected animal, most often bat or monkey

    Contact with infected body fluids from infected person

    Sexual contact

Geographic distribution:

    Ebola: higher incidence in West Africa

    Marburg: seen in parts of southern Africa

DIAGNOSIS

Serology: antibody testing

PCR

Immunohistochemistry

TREATMENT

Supportive

Explanation: This woman has Ebola caused by the Ebola virus. This infection is mainly seen in West Africa. Ebola infections may start as a febrile illness with constitutional symptoms; eventually, diarrhea and gastrointestinal symptoms may be seen. Finally, hemorrhagic fever may occur. Infections are usually diagnosed with serology and molecular methodologies.

Micro gem: EBV and ●48, Cytomegalovirus (CMV) ● may both cause infectious mononucleosis. The heterophile antibody is positive for EBV mononucleosis but negative for CMV mononucleosis.

Vignette: A 16-year-old boy visits his primary care physician with a 4-day history of a sore throat, fever, and general malaise. He states that he is very tired and just wants to sleep. His mother notes that he has not been eating as much as he normally does. His medical history is unremarkable, and he is not on any medication. Upon examination, notable pharyngeal inflammation and white tonsillar exudate is observed. In addition, he has marked posterior cervical lymphadenopathy. His temperature at the time of the examination is 38.8°C (101.8°F). A CBC demonstrates the presence of atypical lymphocytes.

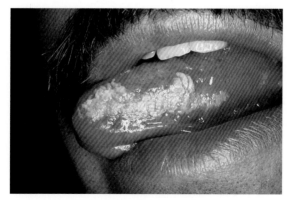

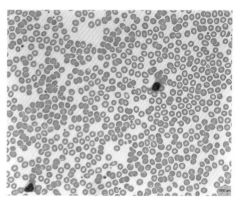

(1) *Source:* CDC/J.S. Greenspan, B.D.S., University of California, San Francisco; Sol Silverman, Jr., D.D.S
CDC public health library PHIL (phil.cdc.gov) image No. 6061
(http://phil.cdc.gov/phil/details_linked.asp?pid=6061)

(2) *Source:* User: Dr Erhabor Osro (own work) [CC BY-SA 3.0 (http://creativecommons.org/licenses/by-sa/3.0)], via Wikimedia Commons, "Atypical lymphocytes a common finding in viral infections." (Retrieved on July 5, 2016 from https://commons.wikimedia.org/wiki/File:Atypical_lymphocytes_2.jpg)

51 Epstein-Barr virus (EBV)

DESCRIPTION

Taxonomy: Herpesvirus family
See also ● 48, Cytomegalovirus (CMV)●; ● 139, Herpes simplex virus (HSV)-1 and -2●; ● 52, Human herpes virus-6 (HHV-6)●; ● 117, Varicella-zoster virus ●
Virus properties: double-stranded DNA, enveloped
Also called human herpes virus-4

INFECTIONS
PRIMARY

Many infections are subclinical
Systemic: infectious mononucleosis—classic symptoms include pharyngitis with exudate, lymphadenopathy
Head and neck: oral cavity—oral hairy leukoplakia (1) in HIV patients

PATHOGENESIS

Target cell is mainly B lymphocytes
May remain latent in B cells

EPIDEMIOLOGY

Transmission: mainly saliva
Most common cause of infectious mononucleosis
Infectious mononucleosis typically infects adolescents and young adults
EBV is associated with nasopharyngeal carcinoma, Burkitt's lymphoma and other malignancies

DIAGNOSIS

Serology: antibody testing—detection of antibodies to viral capsid antigen, nuclear antigen, or early D antigen
For infectious mononucleosis, heterophile antibody is positive—not specific for EBV
CBC: atypical lymphocytes (2) may be present—not specific for EBV

TREATMENT

Mainly supportive
Acyclovir for some cases such as oral hairy leukoplakia

Explanation: Epstein-Barr virus is a herpes virus and a double-stranded DNA virus. EBV may present as pharyngitis with severe lethargy. Often atypical lymphocytes are present in the peripheral blood. Another test of historical importance is the heterophile antibody test. The heterophile antibody is a nonspecific antibody that reacts with EBV.

Vignette: A previously healthy 7-month-old girl presents with a 2-day history of fever and runny nose. The mother states that the baby has been fussier than normal but is feeding normally. The baby attends day care. The girl's temperature is 39.8°C (103.6°F), and her physical exam is unremarkable. The mother is instructed to manage the fever with Tylenol and return if the fever continues. Within a day, the mother notes that the fever has disappeared but the baby now has a small rash on her stomach and back. Within a few days the rash is gone.

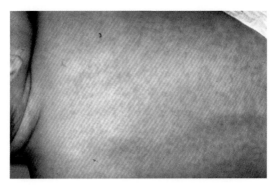

(1) Source: http://medicine.academic.ru/81882/exanthema_subitum.

52 Human herpes virus-6 (HHV-6)

DESCRIPTION

Taxonomy: Herpesvirus family; *Roseolovirus* genus
See also ● 48, Cytomegalovirus (CMV) ●; ● 51, Epstein-Barr virus (EBV) ●; ● 139, Herpes simplex virus (HSV)-1 and -2 ●; ● 117, Varicella-zoster virus ●
Virus properties: double-stranded DNA, enveloped

INFECTIONS

Roseola infantum also called exanthem subitum and sixth disease

PRIMARY

Systemic: constitutional symptoms with high fever—seizures may occur due to the high fever
Skin: exanthem (follows fever)—maculopapular, blanching rash (1); nonpruritic; starts at trunk and moves to face and extremities

OTHER

Complications (rare—most cases are self-limiting)
Nervous: meningitis, encephalitis

EPIDEMIOLOGY

Transmission: secretions, mainly saliva
Peak age of infection: 6 to 12 months

DIAGNOSIS

Usually based on clinical findings

TREATMENT

Supportive

Explanation: This child most likely has roseola infantum. The etiologic agent of this infection is most often human herpes virus-6 (HHV-6), but other viruses, such as HHV-7, ● 140, Non-polio enteroviruses ●, ● 31, Parainfluenza virus ●, and ● 18, Adenovirus ●, may also be the causative agent. Infections most often begin with an abrupt onset of high fever followed by the exanthem. Fever may be accompanied by seizures. Two of the main complications are meningitis and encephalitis.

53   Human immunodeficiency virus (HIV)

Vignette: A 36-year-old man presents with extreme fatigue. He works as a flight attendant and recently ended a trip early due to fatigue and "just feeling sick." He is a man who has sex with men and is currently in a monogamous relationship. His temperature is 38.2°C (100.8°F). Physical exam reveals mild pharyngitis without exudate, cervical lymphadenopathy, and a maculopapular rash on his trunk and back. Both screening and confirmatory tests are positive for HIV.

HIV: Viral Structure

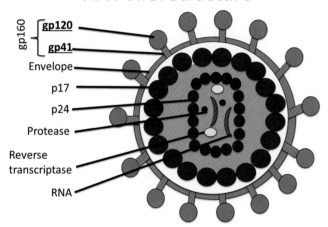

(1)

53 Human immunodeficiency virus (HIV)

DESCRIPTION

Taxonomy: Retrovirus family; *Lentivirus* genus

Virus properties: single-stranded, positive-sense RNA, enveloped (1)

Diploid genome: two identical single-stranded, positive-sense RNA

Human species: HIV-1 and HIV-2

Further classified into groups within each species—HIV-1 group M is most common worldwide (major group)

Group M is further classified into subtypes

INFECTIONS
PRIMARY

HIV/AIDS

Systemic:

Asymptomatic initially

Initial stage (a few months after infection): constitutional symptoms

Latency stage (may last years after initial infection): asymptomatic

Advanced disease (AIDS): < 200 CD4 cells/mm³; opportunistic infections or neoplasms may cause serious disease or death

LIFE CYCLE

1. Viral entry into host cell

Attachment: HIV envelope protein gp120 binds to CD4 on T lymphocytes (and other cell types); gp120 binds to co-receptor CCR5 (mainly on monocytes/macrophages) or CXCR4 (mainly on T lymphocytes)

Fusion of virus and host cell, mediated by viral protein gp41

2. Reverse transcription: viral reverse transcriptase facilitates conversion of single-stranded RNA (ssRNA) into double-stranded DNA (dsDNA)

3. Integration: viral integrase facilitates integration of viral DNA into host DNA (now called provirus)

4. Transcription

5. Translation

6. Viral assembly

7. Viral release (budding) and maturation

EPIDEMIOLOGY

Transmission:

Sexual contact

Parenteral

Vertical: *in utero*, perinatal, and postnatal/breast-feeding

Geographic distribution:

HIV-1: worldwide and is more prevalent

HIV-2: endemic in West Africa, but can also be seen worldwide, including in North America

DIAGNOSIS

Screening test: screens for HIV-1 and HIV-2, antigen (p24) **and** antibody

Most often enzyme-linked immunosorbent assay (ELISA) is used

Confirmatory test: differentiation test for HIV-1 or HIV-2 antibody

Most often chemiluminescent immunoassay is used

If confirmatory test is inconclusive, nucleic acid testing (PCR) must be performed

Viral load (RNA detection and quantification): used for monitoring therapy and infectiousness or as a prognosis indicator

HIV-1 genotype sequencing—aids in predicting resistance patterns

Flow cytometry: for CD4 T-cell levels

TREATMENT

Antiretroviral therapy (ART) or highly active antiretroviral therapy (HAART)

Most often fixed-dose combination of drugs in a single tablet are used.

Usually consists of two nucleotide reverse transcriptase inhibitor plus nonnucleoside RT inhibitor or protease inhibitor or integrase inhibitor

Integrase strand transfer inhibitors—dolutegravir, elvitegravir

Nucleotide RT inhibitor—abacavir, lamivudine, tenofovir

Nonnucleotide RT inhibitor—efavirenz, rilpivirine

Protease inhibitors—atazanavir, darunavir

Other agents: entry inhibitors, fusion inhibitors, reverse transcriptase (RT) inhibitors

Explanation: Primary or acute HIV may present with nonspecific constitutional symptoms and may go unnoticed. Following the initial period, latency occurs. During this time, the infected individual does not usually have manifestations of illness. When the CD4 count drops below 200 cells/mm³, the HIV infection progresses to AIDS. Additionally, opportunistic infections and malignancies occur as the CD4 count decreases.

Vignette: A 37-year-old journalist is in Sierra Leone for 3 months on assignment. One morning he wakes up with a fever and decides to stay home from work. The next day he is still febrile and also experiences chills, malaise, and headache. The following day he decides to visit a local clinic. At that time his temperature is 39.2°C (102.6°F) and he looks visibly ill. His CBC and basic metabolic panel are normal. The clinic physician suspects malaria and orders a thick smear and a thin smear, which are subsequently found to be negative. Reverse transcriptase-polymerase chain reaction (RT-PCR) confirms the diagnosis and demonstrates the presence of a virus.

DESCRIPTION

Taxonomy: Arenavirus family
Virus properties: single-stranded, ambisense RNA, enveloped

INFECTIONS
PRIMARY

Lassa fever
Systemic: febrile illness with maculopapular rash; hemorrhagic form of infection may occur

EPIDEMIOLOGY

Reservoir: rats
Transmission: inhalation, ingestion, or contact with infected animal's secretions
Geographic distribution: higher incidence in West Africa

DIAGNOSIS

Serology: antibody and antigen testing
PCR
Immunohistochemistry—post-mortem

TREATMENT

Supportive

Explanation: Lassa virus may cause a mild febrile illness, such as in this case or a more serious hemorrhagic disease. Infections are endemic in several West African countries, including Sierra Leone, Liberia, and Nigeria. RT-PCR can aid in the diagnosis.

Micro gem: Parvovirus B19 infects RBCs.

Other pathogens that infect RBCs include ●56, *Babesia microti* ●, ●59, *Plasmodium* ●, ●42, *Bartonella* ● (Oroyo fever/Carrion's disease), and ●49, Colorado tick virus ●

Vignette: A 7-year-old girl presents to her pediatrician with a red rash on her cheeks. Her mother states that about 3 days prior, the girl had a fever and runny nose. Other than the erythematous rash on her cheek, her physical examination is unremarkable.

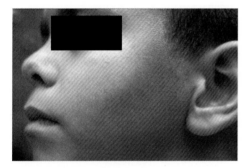

(1) *Source:* CDC/Dr. Philip S. Brachman
CDC public health library PHIL (phil.cdc.gov) image No. 4508
(http://phil.cdc.gov/phil/details_linked.asp?pid=4508)

55 Parvovirus B19

DESCRIPTION

Taxonomy: Parvovirus family
Virus properties: single-stranded DNA, non-enveloped

INFECTIONS
PRIMARY

Postnatal infections
Systemic/skin and soft tissue: erythema infectiosum, also called fifth disease—classic symptoms include flu-like symptoms followed by erythematous maculopapular rash on cheek, resembling a slapped cheek (1)
Musculoskeletal: polyarthritis in adults
Possible complications: aplastic crisis
Congenital: hydrops fetalis, intrauterine fetal death
TORCH = congenital infections
● 14, *Toxoplasma gondii* ●; ● **O**ther (● 106, *Treponema pallidum* ●; ● 117, Varicella-zoster virus ●) ● 142, **R**ubella virus ●; ● 48, **C**ytomegalovirus (CMV) ●; ● 139, **H**erpes simplex virus (HSV)-1 and -2 ●

PATHOGENESIS

Virus infects RBCs
Replication requires that host cell is undergoing DNA replication; virus infects dividing cells such as erythropoietic cells

EPIDEMIOLOGY

Transmission:
Respiratory droplets
Vertical: *in utero*
Infected blood or blood products
Erythema infectiosum is mainly seen in young children
Individuals with sickle cell disease are at risk for aplastic crisis

DIAGNOSIS

Serology: antibody testing
PCR

TREATMENT

Supportive

Explanation: Parvovirus B19, a single-stranded DNA virus, is the causative agent of erythema infectiosum, also called fifth disease. The classic symptom is "slapped cheeks" or an erythematous rash on the cheek. Most often school-aged children present in this manner, whereas adults present with arthralgia. Since this virus infects RBCs, individuals with defects in RBC function, such as sickle cell disease, are at risk for aplastic crisis. If a pregnant woman is infected, she may infect the fetus, leading to severe congenital disease or fetal demise.

Micro gem: *Babesia microti* and ● 125, *Borrelia burgdorferi* ● (Lyme disease) are transmitted by the same vector, the *Ixodes* tick.

Vignette: A 45-year-old man presents to the emergency department with fever and chills of 4 days' duration. He states that he is extremely tired and feels weak. He mentions that about 2 months ago he had been vacationing on Martha's Vineyard, an island off the coast of Massachusetts. At the time of examination his temperature is 39.9°C (103.8°F). His physical exam is unremarkable. A blood smear demonstrates the presence of a ring-shaped structure within his red blood cells.

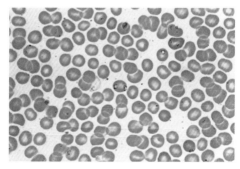

(1) *Source:* CDC/Dr. Mae Melvin
    CDC public health library PHIL (phil.cdc.gov) image No. 10948
    (http://phil.cdc.gov/phil/details_linked.asp?pid=10948)

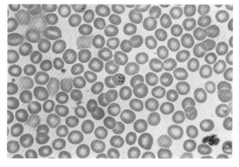

(2) *Source:* CDC/Dr. Mae Melvin
    CDC public health library PHIL (phil.cdc.gov) image No. 11091
    (http://phil.cdc.gov/phil/details_linked.asp?pid=11091)

DESCRIPTION

Protozoa: apicomplexa
Clinically significant morphological forms: ring (1), merozoites (2)

INFECTIONS
PRIMARY

Systemic: fever without periodicity, chills, and malaise

PATHOGENESIS

Parasite infects RBCs

EPIDEMIOLOGY

Transmission: bite of *Ixodes* tick (same vector as *Borrelia burgdorferi*)
Geographic distribution: mostly Northeast U.S (Nantucket Island, Martha's Vineyard) and parts of Midwest U.S.

DIAGNOSIS

Microscopy: identification of parasite from Giemsa stain thick and thin blood smears
 Ring forms (1) or merozoite (2), which resembles a Maltese cross or rosette
PCR
Serology: antibody testing

TREATMENT

Depends on disease severity
 Mild cases: atovaquone plus azithromycin
 Severe cases: clindamycin plus quinine

Explanation: *Babesia* is a parasite that infects red blood cells. It is transmitted to humans via the bite of the tick—the same tick that transmits *Borrelia burgdorferi* (Lyme disease). In the United States, *B. microti* is the most common species, and babesiosis is most often seen in the Northeast. The ring form of the organisms closely resembles ● 59, *Plasmodium* ●. However, the geographic distribution of malaria and babesiosis differs, which aids in the diagnosis.

Vignette: A 21-year-old man in rural Tanzania presents to the clinic with severe swelling of his leg. The swelling has progressively become worse, and he is having difficulty walking. On exam, extreme lymphedema of his right leg is noted, and the skin on the affected leg is hardened. A blood smear stained with Giemsa demonstrates the presence of a microfilaria.

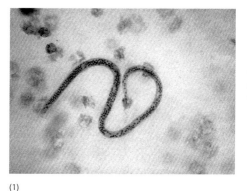

(1)

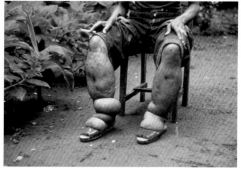

(2) *Source:* CDC public health library PHIL (phil.cdc.gov) image No. 373
(http://phil.cdc.gov/phil/details_linked.asp?pid=373)

DESCRIPTION   Nemathelminth / roundworm: filaria
Clinically significant morphological forms: microfilariae—larvae (1); filariae—adult worms

INFECTIONS
PRIMARY   Lymphatic
Acute: lymphadenopathy
Chronic: lymphedema/elephantiasis (2), usually of lower extremities and genitalia

PATHOGENESIS   Mosquito transmits larvae: larvae develop into adults; adults lay eggs, which mature into larvae; larvae in bloodstream
Adult worms may block lymphatic vessels, resulting in lymphedema

EPIDEMIOLOGY   Transmission: bite of a mosquito (night biting mosquitoes)
Geographic distribution: depends on species
W. bancrofti—mainly Indian subcontinent, sub-Saharan Africa
B. malayi—mainly Southeast Asia

DIAGNOSIS   Microscopy: identification of microfilariae from Giemsa stain blood smears
The number of microfilariae in the blood peak during the night. Hence, blood should be drawn during the night, if possible.
Serology: antigen testing

TREATMENT   Diethylcarbamazine (DEC)

Explanation: Severe lymphedema or elephantiasis is a finding observed in infections with the nematodes *Wuchereria* and *Brugia*. Infections may be asymptomatic or result in acute lymphadenopathy. Chronic infections result in lymphedema, as noted in this case.

Vignette: A 34-year-old woman presents to the emergency department with conjunctivitis and a sensation of foreign body in her left eye. She recently returned from visiting family in Angola. On exam, the infected eye is slightly swollen, and a small worm approximately 40 to 50 mm is seen within the eye on the conjunctiva.

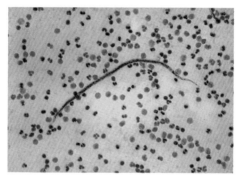

(1) *Source:* CDC/Dr. Lee Moore
CDC public health library PHIL (phil.cdc.gov) image No. 914
(http://phil.cdc.gov/phil/details_linked.asp?pid=914)

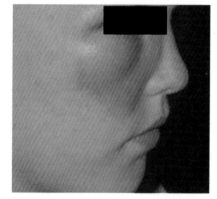

(2) *Source:* J.D. MacLean Centre for Tropical Diseases at McGill

DESCRIPTION
Nemathelminth / roundworm: filaria
Clinically significant morphological forms: microfilariae—larvae (1); filariae—adult worms
Alternative name: African eye worm

INFECTIONS
PRIMARY
Loaiasis
Lymphatic: calabar swelling (subcutaneous tissue swelling) (2)
Head and neck: eye—adult worm migrates to eye (referred to as eye worm)

EPIDEMIOLOGY
Transmission: bite of a deerfly, also called mango fly
Geographic distribution: mainly Central Africa

DIAGNOSIS
Microscopy: identification of microfilaria in blood or tissue
Serology: antibody testing

TREATMENT
Diethylcarbamazine (DEC), albendazole

Explanation: This woman has an infection with the filarial parasite *Loa loa*, which is transmitted by the bite of a deerfly. Infections are mainly seen in Central Africa. Infections are often asymptomatic, but subcutaneous swellings, also referred to as calabar swellings, may be seen, especially on the face and the extremities. Often infections are diagnosed as the worm migrates to eye, which may result in inflammation of the eye and surrounding area.

59 Plasmodium

Micro gem: The ring form of *Plasmodium* looks very similar to the ring form of ●56, *Babesia microti* ●. However, the geographic distribution and vectors of these pathogens are different.

Vignette: A 36-year-old man presents with a 2-week history of periodic fever and myalgia. He works as a photographer, and recently returned from a trip to several African countries. His temperature is 39.2°C (102.6°F), pulse 100, and blood pressure 112/57 mm Hg. On abdominal exam, he has mild tenderness in his left upper quadrant. Giemsa-stained blood smears show a crescent-shaped gametocyte.

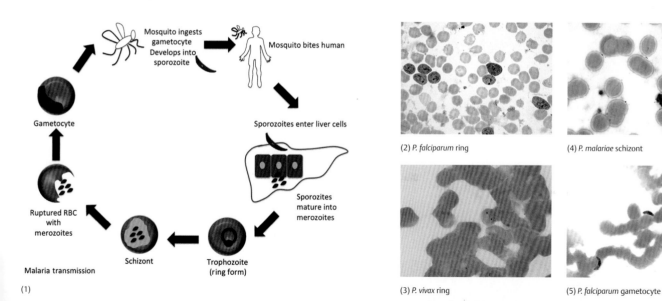

Mosquito ingests gametocyte Develops into sporozoite

Mosquito bites human

Gametocyte

Sporozoites enter liver cells

Ruptured RBC with merozoites

Sporozites mature into merozoites

Schizont

Trophozoite (ring form)

Malaria transmission

(1)

(2) *P. falciparum* ring

(4) *P. malariae* schizont

(3) *P. vivax* ring

(5) *P. falciparum* gametocyte

DESCRIPTION

Protozoa: apicomplexa

Clinically significant morphological forms: ring, trophozoite, schizont with merozoites, gametocyte, hypozoite—seen only in *P. vivax* and *P. ovale*

Clinically important species: *P. falciparum*, *P. vivax*, *P. malariae*, *P. ovale*, *P. knowlesi*

INFECTIONS

PRIMARY

Malaria

Systemic: paroxysms (recurrent episodes) of fever and chills

	Paroxysms	Relapse	Geographic distribution
P. falciparum	Every 48 hours	No	Tropics and subtropics
P. vivax	Every 48 hours	Yes	Tropics and subtropics
P. ovale	Every 48 hours	Yes	Mainly western Africa
P. malariae	Every 72 hours	No	Tropics and subtropics
P. knowlesi	Daily fevers may be seen	No	Mainly Southeast Asia

P. falciparum: secondary sequelae

Nervous: cerebral malaria

Respiratory: respiratory distress

Systemic: anemia (blackwater fever)

PATHOGENESIS

Parasite infects RBCs (1)

P. vivax and *P. ovale* only: hypnozoite remains dormant in liver, leading to relapses

EPIDEMIOLOGY

Transmission: bite of an *Anopheles* mosquito (1)

Geographic distribution: mainly tropical and subtropical countries, especially South and Central America, Africa, Asia, South Pacific, and parts of Middle East

DIAGNOSIS

Microscopy: identification of parasite from Giemsa stained thick and thin blood smears

Evaluate RBC and parasite

RBC: evaluate infected RBC age, size, and shape, RBC inclusions (i.e., Shüffner's dots)

Parasite: evaluate ring form (2,3), schizont and number of merozoites (4) and gametocyte (5)

Characteristic features: *P. malariae*—band-shaped trophozoite, *P. falciparum*—crescent-shaped gametocyte

Rapid assays

TREATMENT

Depends on manifestations, complications and other findings

Chloroquine phosphate, quinine plus doxycycline, mefloquine, artemisinin

For *P. vivax* or *P. ovale*, add primaquine phosphate to target hypnozoites

Conditions that confer resistance or decrease the severity of infection: G6PD deficiency, thalassemia

P. vivax—individuals that are Duffy antigen negative

P. falciparum—individuals with sickle cell hemoglobin

Explanation: The characteristic feature of malaria is paroxysm of fever, which corresponds to the release of the merozoites from the schizont. Malaria is caused by the protozoan parasite *Plasmodium*, and several species are considered human pathogens. In this case the crescent-shaped gametocyte suggests that *P. falciparum* is the causative agent. The ring forms, trophozoites, schizonts, and gametocytes can be seen in Giemsa-stained blood smears.

Vignette 1: A 38-year-old immigrant from Brazil presents with difficulty swallowing and chest pain. Her vitals and physical exam are unremarkable. Chest X-ray shows a dilated esophagus, and a barium swallow reveals narrowing of the esophagus. Manometry demonstrates a nonrelaxing esophageal sphincter and loss of peristaltic movement in the lower esophagus. Serology confirms an infectious etiology.

Vignette 2: A 53-year-old man in Tanzania presents with fever and malaise. He works as a safari tour guide and spends much of his time outdoors. Based on his symptoms he is diagnosed with malaria and treated with chloroquine. He stays home from work with a persistent fever for the next 2 weeks. During this time, he also develops a severe headache and is having difficulty sleeping. Within a few days he is hallucinating and experiencing memory loss. At the hospital his temperature is 38.9°C (102°F). Cerebrospinal fluid (CSF) is obtained and a Giemsa stain shows trypanomastigotes.

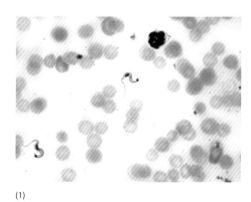

(1)

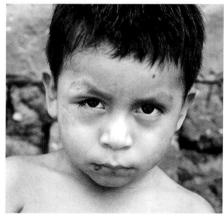

(2) *Source:* CDC/Dr. Mae Melvin
CDC public health library PHIL (phil.cdc.gov) image No. 2617
(http://phil.cdc.gov/phil/details_linked.asp?pid=2617)

DESCRIPTION
Protozoa: flagellate
Clinically significant morphological forms: trypomastigote (C-shaped) (1), amastigote
Clinically significant species: *T. cruzi, T. brucei rhodesiense, T. brucei gambiense*

INFECTIONS
PRIMARY
T. cruzi: Chagas disease
    Systemic: constitutional symptoms
    Head and neck: eye—unilateral swelling of eyelid [Romaña's sign (2)]—*T. cruzi* penetrates through conjunctiva
    Skin and soft tissue: chagoma—*T. cruzi* penetrates through skin
    Secondary sequelae:
        Cardiovascular: cardiomyopathy
        Gastrointestinal: dysphagia, megaesophagus, megacolon
T. b. gambiense and *T. b. rhodesiense:* West and East African sleeping sickness respectively
    Early stage:
        Systemic: constitutional symptoms
        Skin and soft tissue: chancre at bite site
        Lymphatic: lymphadenopathy
    Late stage:
        Nervous: drowsiness, behavioral changes, difficulty walking, slurred speech; coma

EPIDEMIOLOGY
Transmission:
    T. cruzi: reduviid bug also called triatomine bug and kissing bug; vector injects parasite via saliva or defecation while taking a blood meal
    T.b. gambiense and *rhodesiense:* bite of a tsetse fly

Geographic distribution:
    T. cruzi: South and Central America
    T. b. gambiense: West Africa
    T. b. rhodesiense: East Africa

DIAGNOSIS
Microscopy: identification of trypomastigote (1) from Giemsa-stained thick and thin blood smears or cerebrospinal fluid (CSF)
Serology: antibody testing

TREATMENT
Depends on infecting species and clinical stage
Acute stage *T. cruzi:* nifurtimox

Explanation 1: Dysphagia and chest pain are classic symptoms of achalasia in which there is a dilation of the esophagus. Chronic Chagas disease, caused by the protozoan parasite *Trypanosoma cruzi*, may result in heart disease and gastrointestinal disease, including achalasia. Serological testing would confirm that the etiology is *T. cruzi*. Acute infections with *T. cruzi* begin with constitutional symptoms, including fever, malaise, and anorexia. Unilateral swelling of eyelid or Romaña's sign is a characteristic finding during this stage. There is an increased prevalence of *T. cruzi* in South American countries, such as Brazil.

Explanation 2: This man's infection is most likely to be due to *T. brucei gambiense* & *T. b. rhodesiense* the agents of African sleeping sickness. *T. b. rhodesiense* is mainly seen in East Africa and *T. b. gambiense* is mainly seen in West Africa. Both these pathogens are transmitted by the bite of a tsetse fly. The early stage of African sleeping sickness is marked by non-specific constitutional symptoms, development of a chancre at the bite site and lymphadenopathy. During the late stage, the pathogen affects the nervous system resulting in drowsiness, behavioral changes, difficulty walking, slurred speech and eventually coma.

Micro gem: Both *Bacillus cereus* and ● 134, *Staphylococcus aureus* ● cause emetic foodborne illness with short incubation times (< 6 hours).

Vignette: A 46-year-old man suddenly feels ill and starts vomiting at 1 a.m. He continues vomiting two or three times per hour for the next 4 hours. The man had Chinese take-out for dinner the previous evening and had consumed vegetable fried rice and beef lo mein. By the next afternoon he is feeling better.

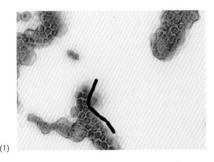

(1)

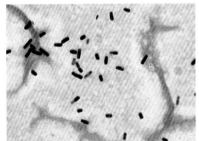

(2)

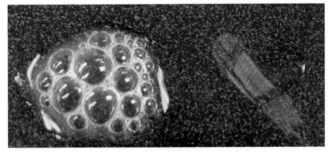

(3) Catalase Test. Left side, catalase positive. Right side, catalase negative.

61   *Bacillus cereus*

DESCRIPTION
Gram-positive rods (1,2) large, flattened ends
Spore-producer

INFECTIONS
PRIMARY
Gastrointestinal: emetic (< 6 hours incubation), diarrheal—watery diarrhea (10- to 12-hour incubation)

OTHER
Head and neck: eye—endophthalmitis, keratitis
Skin and soft tissue/musculoskeletal: wounds

PATHOGENESIS
Enterotoxins
Heat stable (ST): emetic toxin—preformed in food
Heat labile (LT): diarrheal toxin—increases cAMP—toxin is formed *in vivo*
See also ●68, Enteroxigenic *Escherichia coli* ●; ●73, *Vibrio cholerae* ●; ●23, *Bordetella pertussis* ●; ●109, *Bacillus anthracis* ●

EPIDEMIOLOGY
Transmission:
GI infections — foodborne
Emetic—commonly associated foods include starchy foods, such as fried rice and potatoes;
Diarrheal—commonly associated foods include meats and cream sauces
Eye and skin infections: eye or skin inoculation following penetrating trauma

DIAGNOSIS
Usually made on clinical and epidemiological findings
Culture: catalase positive (3), beta-hemolytic

TREATMENT
GI infections: none recommended; self-limiting
Other infection types: vancomycin, clindamycin

Explanation: This man has an infection due to the emetic toxin of *Bacillus cereus*. *B. cereus* causes two types of foodborne illness: emetic and diarrheal. The emetic illness has a short incubation phase (usually < 6 hours) and is associated with starchy foods, such as potatoes and rice. When rice is left out at room temperature, the sporulated organism germinates and produces the toxin. When the rice is re-heated, such as the case with fried rice, the toxin, which is heat stable, remains viable and can then be transmitted to humans. Diarrheal disease with this pathogen is very similar to foodborne infections with ●110, *Clostridium perfringens* ● and is caused by a heat-labile toxin.

Micro gem: *Campylobacter,* ●73, *Vibrio* ●, and ●69, *Helicobacter* ● are clinically significant curved gram-negative rods

Vignette: A 40-year-old woman presents to the emergency department with diarrhea and severe abdominal pain. She has had six or seven bowel movements per day for the past 3 days, and during the last 24 hours she has noticed blood in her stool. She states she had a fever and felt "flu-like" the first day of her illness but does not feel like that anymore. She had attended a family picnic one week ago and had eaten grilled chicken. At the time of the examination, her temperature is 37.2° C (99.0° F). Physical examination reveals abdominal tenderness. The stool culture grows a pathogen on selective media at 42°C.

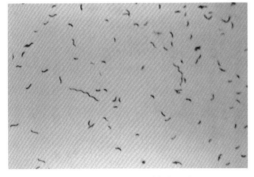
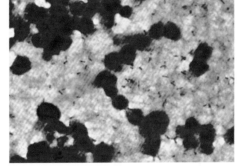

(1) *Source:* CDC public health library PHIL (phil.cdc.gov) image No. 6657
(http://phil.cdc.gov/phil/details_linked.asp?pid=6657)

(2)

DESCRIPTION Gram-negative rods, curved, comma-, seagull-, or S-shaped (1)

INFECTIONS

PRIMARY Gastrointestinal: enteritis or colitis—watery diarrhea; bloody diarrhea; dysentery-like illness with tenesmus, fever may be present

OTHER Postinfectious sequelae
Musculoskeletal: reactive arthritis
Nervous: Guillain-Barré syndrome

PATHOGENESIS Invasion and inflammation of mucosa: may cause histological damage to mucosal surface
Guillain-Barré due to cross-reactive antibodies (*C. jejuni* antibodies cross-react with gangliosides)

EPIDEMIOLOGY Transmission:
Most common: foodborne—commonly associated foods include poultry and unpasteurized milk
Rare: contact with infected animals—commonly associated animals include dogs, cats, poultry, sheep, and cattle
Rare: person-to-person via fecal-oral route

DIAGNOSIS Culture: growth on selective media, oxidase positive, microaerophilic, capnophilic, growth at 42°C
Fecal leukocytes may be positive (2)
PCR from stool

TREATMENT Mostly self-limiting; severe cases—azithromycin

Explanation: *Campylobacter* enteritis may be indistinguishable from infections with ● 70, Nontyphoidal *Salmonella* ●, ● 71, *Shigella* ●, and ● 74, *Yersinia enterocolitica* and *pseudotuberculosis* ●. Bloody diarrhea may be present, as in this case. The pathogen is transmitted via ingestion of contaminated food, especially undercooked poultry and unpasteurized milk. *Campylobacter* is a curved gram-negative rod that grows well at 42°C on selective media in microaerophilic and capnophilic conditions. It is one of the most common causes of bacterial gastroenteritis worldwide.

Micro gem: *C. difficile* is a common health-care associated pathogen and is associated with antibiotic use.

Vignette: A 54-year-old woman is in the hospital recovering from a surgical procedure. She develops watery diarrhea and a fever. She is on several medications including clindamycin. Her temperature is 38.3°C (100.9°F). A CBC demonstrates a leukocyte count of 18.3 × 10⁹/L. A PCR from a stool specimen is positive for *C. difficile* toxin A and B.

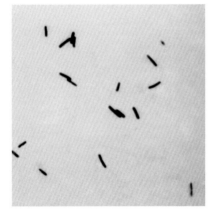

(1) *Source:* CDC/Dr. Holdeman
CDC public health library PHIL (phil.cdc.gov) image
No. 3648
(http://phil.cdc.gov/phil/details_linked.asp?pid=3648)

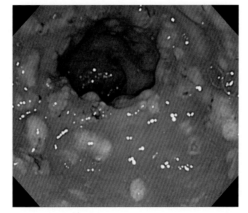

(2) *Source:* Pseudomembranous colitis 1, User: Samir (own work)
[CC BY-SA 3.0 (http://creativecommons.org/licenses/
by-sa/3.0)], via Wikimedia Commons
(https://upload.wikimedia.org/wikipedia/commons/d/dc/
Pseudomembranous_colitis_1.jpg)

63 *Clostridium difficile*

DESCRIPTION
Gram-positive rods (1), large, boxcar shaped
Spore-producer
Obligate anaerobe

INFECTIONS
PRIMARY
Gastrointestinal: asymptomatic carrier; colitis—watery diarrhea, mucus may be present; pseudomembranous colitis (2); fulminant colitis; recurrent infections may occur

PATHOGENESIS
Enterotoxins:
 C. difficile toxin (CDT) A—recruits PMNs, disrupts tight junctions, increases permeability of intestinal wall, induces inflammation
 CDT B—cytotoxin that disrupts cytoskeleton, depolymerizes actin; essential for virulence

EPIDEMIOLOGY
May be part of GI microbiota
Transmission:
 Fecal-oral (ingestion of spores)
 Fomites
 Displacement of endogenous strains (less common)
Nosocomial pathogen
Risk factor: antibiotic use; frequently associated with fluoroquinolones, clindamycin, penicillins, and cephalosporins

DIAGNOSIS
Toxin detection by PCR or EIA
EIA for glutamate dehydrogenase (GDH)
Cell culture for cytotoxicity (not frequently utilized anymore)

PREVENTION
C. difficile spores are alcohol-resistant: vigorously wash hands with soap and water instead of hand sanitizer to eliminate spores
Patient's with *C. difficile* are placed on contact precautions while in the hospital
Fecal transplant: may prevent recurrent infections

TREATMENT
Discontinue broad-spectrum antibiotics
Effective agents include metronidazole, oral vancomycin; recurrent infections—fidaxomicin, rifaximin

ANIMATION
http://go.thieme.com/microb/Video63.1

Explanation: *Clostridium difficile* is an agent of watery diarrhea and pseudomembranous colitis. Recurrent infections, in which there is a relapse of infection with *C. difficile,* are problematic. Additionally, individuals may be asymptomatic carriers or have more serious manifestations such as fulminant colitis. *C. difficile*, an anaerobic gram-positive rod, produces endospores and two exotoxins (toxin A and toxin B). Infections are often health-care associated, and antibiotic use increases the risk of infection with this pathogen.

Vignette: While vising Thailand, a 21-year-old woman suddenly develops diarrhea. She has been in the country for about 1 week and frequents the local street venders. The woman has four or five bowel movements per day, and the stool appears watery with no apparent blood. Within a few days, she is feeling better.

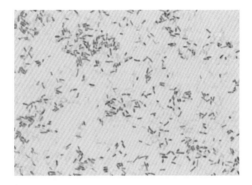

(1)

DESCRIPTION

Gram-negative rods (1); part of *Enterobacteriaceae* family
See also ● 103, *Klebsiella granulomatis* ●; ● 131, *Klebsiella pneumoniae* ●; ● 97, *Proteus* ●; ● 47, *Salmonella enterica* serotype typhi and paratyphi ●; ● 70, Nontyphoidal *Salmonella* ●; ● 71, *Shigella* ●; ● 74, *Yersinia enterocolitica and pseudotuberculosis* ●; ● 138, *Yersinia pestis* ●

INFECTIONS
 PRIMARY

Gastrointestinal: enteritis—infant diarrhea, traveler's diarrhea; both present as watery diarrhea

PATHOGENESIS

Fimbriae: tight adherence
Enterotoxin:
 EAST—heat stable toxin that binds to guanylate cyclase and increases cyclic guanosine monophosphate (cCGMP) (similar to the ST of ● 68, enterotoxigenic *Escherichia coli* [ETEC] ●)

EPIDEMIOLOGY

Transmission: contaminated food and water
Geographic distribution: mainly seen in resource-limited countries

DIAGNOSIS

Culture not useful; indistinguishable from other *E. coli* in culture
PCR

TREATMENT

Supportive

Explanation: There are several types of *E. coli* that are agents of diarrheal disease. These include EAEC, enteropathogenic *E. coli* (EPEC), enterohemorrhagic *E. coli* (EHEC), enteroinvasive *E. coli* (EIEC), and enterotoxigenic *E. coli* (ETEC). All except EHEC and EIEC cause watery diarrhea. EAEC and ETEC are common agents of traveler's diarrhea, as presented in this case, and it may be difficult to distinguish between these two pathogens based solely on clinical manifestations. EHEC, specifically *E. coli* O157:H7, can be identified by culture using MacConkey agar with sorbitol. It is not possible to distinguish the rest of the GI *E. coli* strains from one another with standard culture techniques.

Vignette: A 5-year-old boy presents to the emergency department with bloody diarrhea of 2 days' duration. His mother reports that earlier that week the family had attended a picnic, and the boy had eaten several hamburgers. At the time of the examination his temperature is 38.9°C (102.0°F). The stool culture is negative for parasites. After 2 days, the bacterial culture grows sorbitol-negative, gram-negative rods.

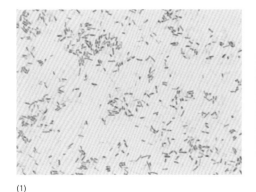

(1)

MacConkey agar. Left side, lactose positive. Right side, lactose negative.

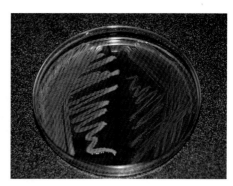

(3) MacConkey with Sorbitol. Left side, sorbitol positive. right side Sorbitol negative.

DESCRIPTION

Gram-negative rods (1); part of family *Enterobacteriaceae*
See also ●103, *Klebsiella granulomatis* ●; ●131, *Klebsiella pneumoniae* ●; ●97, *Proteus* ●; ●47, *Salmonella enterica* serotype typhi and paratyphi ●; ●70, Nontyphoidal *Salmonella* ●; ●71, *Shigella* ●; ●74, *Yersinia enterocolitica and pseudotuberculosis* ●; ●138, *Yersinia pestis* ●
Also called shiga-toxin producing *E. coli* (STEC)
E. coli O157:H7 is a common serotype of EHEC in the U.S.

INFECTIONS

PRIMARY

Gastrointestinal: enteritis—initially watery diarrhea that develops into bloody diarrhea

OTHER

Complication of GI infections
Renal: hemolytic-uremic syndrome (HUS)—anemia, thrombocytopenia, renal failure

PATHOGENESIS

Enterotoxin: verotoxin/Shiga-like toxin—cleaves 28S RNA of 60S ribosome and inhibits protein synthesis (similar to ●71, *Shigella* ●)

EPIDEMIOLOGY

Transmission:
Most common: foodborne—ingestion of the bacteria which produces toxin *in vivo*—commonly associated foods include undercooked ground beef, unpasteurized milk
Person-to-person via fecal-oral route
Rare: contact with infected animals
Low-dose organism (< 100 organisms may cause disease)

DIAGNOSIS

Culture: lactose positive (2), *E. coli* O157:H7 is sorbitol negative on MacConkey with sorbitol agar (different from other *E. coli*) (3)
PCR from stool

TREATMENT

Supportive

ANIMATION

http://go.thieme.com/microb/Video65.1

Explanation: *E. coli* O157:H7 is a gram-negative rod that is part of the *Enterobacteriaceae* family. This pathogen is most often foodborne, and is associated with undercooked beef and other foods. EHEC produces the Shiga-like toxin, which inhibits the 28S ribosome and protein synthesis. One of the laboratory characteristics that can distinguish this pathogen from other *E. coli* strains is that *E. coli* O157:H7 is sorbitol-negative on MacConkey with sorbitol agar. Some patients, especially children, can develop HUS. Clinical manifestations of HUS may include pallor and hematuria. Schistocytes, fragmented red blood cells, may be seen in peripheral blood smears in HUS.

Vignette: A 19-year-old man presents with a 3-day history of fever, abdominal pain, vomiting, and diarrhea. He states that it hurts when he has a bowel movement. He sought medical attention when he noticed blood and mucus in his stool. He mentions that he returned from a spring break trip to Belize a week ago and had eaten food from a street vendor. His temperature is 38.8° C (101.8° F). Stool is collected for laboratory analysis. The ova and parasite examination is negative. The stool is positive for fecal leukocytes.

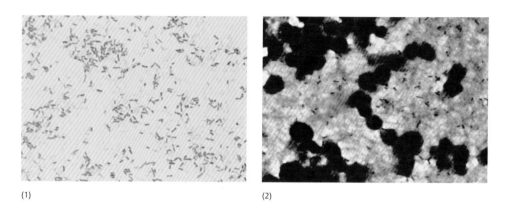

(1)   (2)

66 Enteroinvasive *Escherichia coli* (EIEC)

DESCRIPTION

Gram-negative rods (1); part of *Enterobacteriaceae* family
See also ● 103, *Klebsiella granulomatis* ●; ● 131, *Klebsiella pneumoniae* ●; ● 97, *Proteus* ●; ● 47, *Salmonella enterica* serotype typhi and paratyphi ●; ● 70, Nontyphoidal *Salmonella* ●; ● 71, *Shigella* ●; ● 74, *Yersinia enterocolitica* and *pseudotuberculosis* ●; ● 138, *Yersinia pestis* ●

INFECTIONS
PRIMARY

Gastrointestinal: enteritis or colitis—watery diarrhea, bloody diarrhea, or dysentery, fever may be present

PATHOGENESIS

Invasion of M cells; propels itself through cell cytoplasm by assembly of actin tail—similar to ● 71, *Shigella* ●; ultimately results in inflammation

EPIDEMIOLOGY

Transmission: contaminated food and water
Geographic distribution: mainly in seen in resource-limited countries

DIAGNOSIS

Culture not useful; indistinguishable from other *E. coli* in culture
Fecal leukocytes are often positive (2)
PCR from stool

TREATMENT

Similar to *Shigella*

ANIMATION

http://go.thieme.com/microb/Video66.1

Explanation: Manifestations of dysentery include frequent bowel movements with the presence of mucus and blood in the stool, fever, fecal urgency and tenesmus, and abdominal pain. The infection in this case may be due to *Shigella* or Enteroinvasive *E. col* (EIEC). *S. flexneri* and *S. dysenteriae* are more common outside of the United States and may be seen in travelers. EIEC has an identical mechanism of pathogenesis as *Shigella*, and infections with these pathogens may be difficult to distinguish from one another.

Vignette: A 13-month-old boy in Ghana develops watery diarrhea. His mother brings him to the village clinic when she notices that he is less active than normal. On examination, the child is restless and irritable. He is afebrile, his eyes appear slightly sunken, and skin turgor is poor.

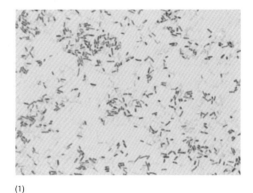

(1)

DESCRIPTION Gram-negative rods (1); part of *Enterobacteriaceae* family
See also ●103, *Klebsiella granulomatis* ●; ●131, *Klebsiella pneumoniae* ●; ●97, *Proteus* ●; ●47, *Salmonella enterica* serotype typhi and paratyphi ●; ●70, Nontyphoidal *Salmonella* ●; ●71, *Shigella* ●; ●74, *Yersinia enterocolitica* and *pseudotuberculosis* ●; ●138, *Yersinia pestis* ●

INFECTIONS
 PRIMARY Gastrointestinal: enteritis—infant diarrhea (watery diarrhea with vomiting)

PATHOGENESIS Attachment: bundle forming pili
Effacement: flattens microvilli and forms pedestals

EPIDEMIOLOGY Transmission:
  Contaminated food and water
  Person-to-person via fecal-oral route
Geographic distribution: mainly seen in resource-limited countries

DIAGNOSIS Culture not useful: indistinguishable from other *E. coli* in culture
PCR from stool

TREATMENT Antimicrobials may shorten course of infection; specific agent will vary based on clinical setting

ANIMATION http://go.thieme.com/microb/Video67.1

Explanation: There are several pathogens that are agents of infant diarrhea in developing nations, including (but not limited to) ●71, *Shigella* ●, ●62, *Campylobacter jejuni* ●, ●68, Enterotoxigenic *Escherichia coli* ● (ETEC), and Enteropathogenic *Escherichia coli* (EPEC). ETEC and EPEC infections result in watery diarrhea as presented here. It would be difficult to identify the exact pathogen in this case without molecular analysis. EPEC should be included in the differential for watery diarrhea in infants in resource-limited countries.

Vignette: A group of college students returns from spring break in Cancun, Mexico, with diarrhea. The diarrhea is watery, and all the students deny fever and the presence of blood in the stool. The students had all consumed lemonade iced tea.

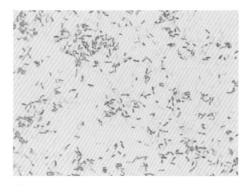

(1)

DESCRIPTION

Gram-negative rods (1); part of *Enterobacteriaceae* family
See also ●103, *Klebsiella granulomatis* ●; ●131, *Klebsiella pneumoniae* ●; ●97, *Proteus* ●; ●47, *Salmonella enterica* serotype typhi and paratyphi ●; ●70, Nontyphoidal *Salmonella* ●; ●71, *Shigella* ●; ●74, *Yersinia enterocolitica* and *pseudotuberculosis* ●; ●138, *Yersinia pestis* ●

INFECTIONS
PRIMARY

Gastrointestinal: enteritis—traveler's diarrhea, infant diarrhea (both present as watery diarrhea)

PATHOGENESIS

Enterotoxins:
Heat-labile toxin (LT): ADP-ribosylates Gs protein and activates adenylate cyclase resulting in increased cAMP (similar to cholera toxin)
See also ●23, *Bordetella pertussis* ●; ●61, *Bacillus cereus* ●; ●73, *Vibrio cholerae* ●; ●109, *Bacillus anthracis* ●
Heat-stable toxin (ST): binds to guanylate cyclase and increases cGMP (similar to EAST of ●64, Enteroaggregative *Escherichia coli* (EAEC) ●)

EPIDEMIOLOGY

Transmission: contaminated food and water
Geographic distribution: mainly seen in resource-limited countries

DIAGNOSIS

Culture not useful—indistinguishable from other *E. coli* in culture
Toxin detection
PCR from stool

TREATMENT

Supportive

ANIMATION

http://go.thieme.com/microb/Video68.1

Explanation: Several pathogens are associated with traveler's diarrhea, including *E. coli* strains, especially Enterotoxigenic *E. coli* (ETEC). This pathogen produces two toxins. The heat-labile toxin is similar in activity to the cholera toxin and increases cAMP, and the heat-stable toxin increases cGMP. The end result of these toxins is watery diarrhea. ETEC is also an agent of diarrhea in infants in resource-limited countries. It is difficult to distinguish infections with ETEC from other GI *E. coli* strains, and pathogen identification must be done with molecular methodology.

Micro gem: Urease is a key pathogenesis factor for *Helicobacter pylori*. Other urease producing pathogens include ●97, **P**roteus mirabilis ●, ●104, *Mycoplasma* and **U**reaplasma ●, ●**N**ocardia ●, and ●11, **C**ryptococcus neoformans and *gatti* ● (PUNCH = urease positive organisms). Note: Only *Ureaplasma*, not *Mycoplasma*, is urease positive.

Vignette: A 45-year-old woman presents to her primary care physician complaining of abdominal pain that had been worsening for the past 2 weeks. She states she also has frequent indigestion, nausea and vomiting, and lack of appetite. Her vitals are unremarkable. Physical examination reveals mild midepigastric tenderness. She denies diarrhea and blood in her stool. A stool antigen for *H. pylori* is positive.

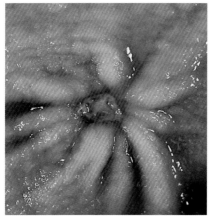

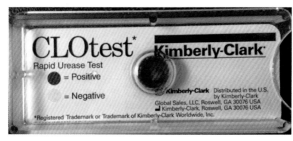

(2)

(1) *Source:* Wikipedia (public domain)
Ed Uthman, MD
(https://en.wikipedia.org/wiki/Timeline_of_peptic_
ulcer_disease_and_Helicobacter_pylori#/media/File:
Benign_gastric_ulcer_1.jpg)

DESCRIPTION Gram-negative rods, spiral, curved

INFECTIONS
PRIMARY Gastrointestinal: peptic ulcer disease (PUD)—acute or chronic gastritis (1), peptic and duodenal ulcers; associated with increased risk of gastric carcinoma and gastric mucosa-associated lymphoid tissue (MALT) lymphoma

PATHOGENESIS Flagella
Adhesins
Urease: breaks down urea and produces ammonia; neutralizes gastric acid
vacA: tissue-damaging cytotoxin
cagA: interferes with epithelial cytoskeleton and induces inflammation

EPIDEMIOLOGY Colonizes stomach of 50% of population
Transmission: most likely fecal-oral

DIAGNOSIS Endoscopy: urease detection via the *Campylobacter*-like organism (CLO) test (2)
Microscopy: histopathology of biopsy
Urea breath test
Serology: serum antibody testing and stool antigen testing

TREATMENT Antibiotic (metronidazole, tinidazole) plus bismuth plus proton pump inhibitor for two weeks

ANIMATION http://go.thieme.com/microb/Video69.1

Explanation: *Helicobacter pylori* is associated with gastric and duodenal ulcers. The most common manifestation is dyspepsia as in this case. *H. pylori* is a curved gram-negative rod. There are several methods for diagnosis. The least invasive tests include stool antigen and breath testing for urease activity. Endoscopy may be performed as well; however, it is more invasive. Serology is not useful for initial diagnosis, as *H. pylori* IgG is present in individuals with past infections as well as current infections.

Micro gem: Typical bacterial stool cultures test for ●70, Nontyphoidal *Salmonella* ●, ●71, *Shigella* ●, ●62, *Campylobacter* ●, and ●65, Enterohemorrhagic *Escherichia coli* (EHEC) ●. If other stool pathogens are suspected, the clinical microbiology laboratory must be notified so appropriate testing can be performed.

Vignette: A 25-year-old woman presents with a 3-day history of fever, abdominal cramps, diarrhea, and vomiting. She denies hematochezia. She states that about 5 days ago she ate an entire batch of uncooked cookie dough. Her temperature is 38.6°C (101.5°F). Physical examination revealed mild abdominal tenderness. The stool culture grew a lactose-negative, H_2S-positive organism on Hektoen agar.

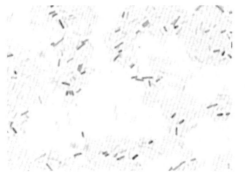

(1)

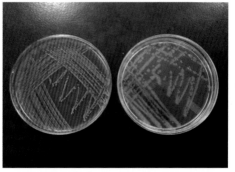
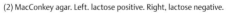

(2) MacConkey agar. Left. lactose positive. Right, lactose negative.

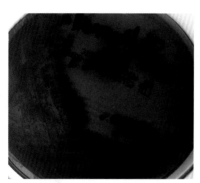

(3) Hektoen agar

DESCRIPTION

Gram-negative rods (1); part of *Enterobacteriaceae* family
See also ●103, *Klebsiella granulomatis* ●; ●131, *Klebsiella pneumoniae* ●; ●97, *Proteus* ●; ●47, *Salmonella enterica* serotype typhi and paratyphi ●; ●71, *Shigella* ●; ●74, *Yersinia enterocolitica* and *pseudotuberculosis* ●; ●138, *Yersinia pestis* ●
Clinically significant species: *S. enterica*; many serotypes—based on O and H antigens
Important serotypes: *S. enterica* serotype Enteritidis, *S. enterica* serotype Typhimurium, *S. enterica* serotype Choleraesuis

INFECTION

PRIMARY

Gastrointestinal: enteritis—most often watery diarrhea; bloody diarrhea or dysentery may be present; fever may be present
Complication of GI infection: dissemination

OTHER

Post-infectious sequelae: reactive arthritis, osteomyelitis

PATHOGENESIS

LPS
Flagella
Adherence: causes membrane ruffling of cell
Invasion and replication in enterocytes and M cells: results in inflammation

EPIDEMIOLOGY

Transmission:
Most common: foodborne—commonly associated foods include poultry, eggs and dairy products
Contact with contaminated animals: commonly associated animals include reptiles
Rare: person-to-person via fecal-oral route
Osteomyelitis associated with individuals with sickle cell disease

DIAGNOSIS

Culture: lactose negative (2), hydrogen sulfide (H$_2$S) positive (3)
PCR from stool

TREATMENT

Supportive
Severe cases: ciprofloxacin, levofloxacin

ANIMATION

http://go.thieme.com/microb/Video70.1

Explanation: Nontyphoidal *Salmonella* is one the leading causes of foodborne diarrhea in the United States. Most often the pathogen is transmitted via contaminated food, such as undercooked poultry and poultry products, including eggs. This woman may have consumed raw eggs in the cookie dough leading to her symptoms. *Salmonella* is a gram-negative rod that grows well on enteric agar such as MacConkey and Hektoen. It is lactose negative and H$_2$S positive.

Micro gem: *Shigella*, ● 66, Enteroinvasive *Escherichia coli* (EIEC) ●, and ● 3, *Listeria monocytogenes* ● invade the host cell then propel themselves through the cell cytoplasm by assembly of an actin tail.

Vignette: A 2-year-old boy presents to the pediatrician with a 2-day history of fever and watery diarrhea. His mother states she was concerned when she saw blood in his diaper. She also mentions that her son attends day care and several other children are also sick with similar symptoms. His temperature is 38.9° C (102.0° F). Stool is collected for laboratory analysis. The ova and parasite examination and the rotavirus EIA are negative. The fecal leukocytes are positive, and the stool culture grows a lactose negative organism on MacConkey agar.

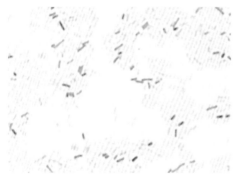

(1)

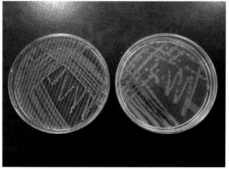

(2) MacConkey agar. Left. lactose positive. Right, lactose negative.

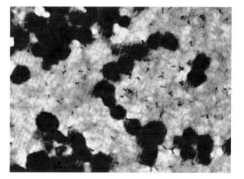

(3)

71 Shigella

DESCRIPTION

Gram-negative rods (1); part of *Enterobacteriaceae* family
See also ● 129, *Escherichia coli* ●; ● 103, *Klebsiella granulomatis* ●; ● 131, *Klebsiella pneumoniae* ●; ● 97, *Proteus* ●; ● 47, *Salmonella enterica* serotype typhi and paratyphi ●; ● 70, Nontyphoidal *Salmonella* ●; ● 74, *Yersinia enterocolitica* and *pseudotuberculosis* ●; ● 138, *Yersinia pestis* ●
Clinically significant species/serotypes: group A—*S. dysenteriae*, group B—*S. flexneri*, group C—*S. boydii*, group D—*S. sonnei*

INFECTIONS

PRIMARY

Gastrointestinal: enteritis or bacillary dysentery—depends on species; ranges from watery or bloody diarrhea; fever in dysentery cases; complication: *S. dysenteriae*—HUS (less common than with Enterohemorrhagic *E. coli*)

OTHER

Post-infectious sequelae: reactive arthritis

PATHOGENESIS

LPS
Invasion and replication in M cells of Peyer's patches in colon causing inflammation (similar to EIEC); propels itself through cell cytoplasm by assembly of actin tail
S. dysenteriae type 1: enterotoxin—Shiga toxin (STX); cleaves 28S RNA of 60S ribosome and disrupts protein synthesis (similar to ● 65, Enterohemorrhagic *Escherichia coli* (EHEC) ●)

EPIDEMIOLOGY

Solely a human pathogen
Transmission:
 Person-to-person via fecal-oral route, ingestion of contaminated food or water

Geographic distribution:
 S. sonnei is the most common species in the U.S.
 S. dysenteriae causes the most severe disease, but is not common in U.S.
Low-dose organism—10 organisms may cause disease
High risk: elderly, young children; epidemics commonly occur in close quarters, such as day care centers and in unsanitary conditions

DIAGNOSIS

Culture: lactose negative (2)
Fecal leukocytes often positive (3)
PCR from stool

TREATMENT

Ciprofloxacin, levofloxacin

ANIMATIONS

http://go.thieme.com/microb/Video71.1;
http://go.thieme.com/microb/Video71.2

Explanation: In the United States, shigellosis is predominately caused by *Shigella sonnei,* and the very young and the elderly at high risk for infections. Although *Shigella* is classically associated with bacillary dysentery, the presentation may vary based on the infecting species. Infections may closely resemble infection with ● 62, *Campylobacter jejuni* ● or ● 70, Nontyphoidal *Salmonella* ●. *Shigella* is a gram-negative, lactose-negative rod.

Vignette: A 23-year-old man presents to the emergency department with a "sore" on his right leg. He had recently gone surfing with friends in southern California and reports that his leg had been injured in the water. His vitals are normal. On examination, an approximately 4-cm circular wound is seen on his right leg. The wound is shallow and red in color, and a small amount of pus is evident. Gram stain from the purulent material reveals curved gram-negative rods.

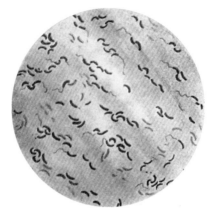

(1) *Source:* CDC public health library PHIL (phil.cdc.gov)
image No. 5324
(http://phil.cdc.gov/phil/details_linked.asp?pid=5324)

DESCRIPTION
Gram-negative rods, curved or comma-shaped (1)
Clinically significant species: *V. vulnificus, V. parahaemolyticus*

INFECTIONS
PRIMARY
Gastrointestinal (GI): watery diarrhea; fever may be present
Skin and soft tissue: wound infections

OTHER
Systemic: bacteremia

PATHOGENESIS
V. vulnificus: exotoxin with protease activity; iron acquisition system

EPIDEMIOLOGY
Halotolerant: associated with salt or brackish water
Transmission:
GI infections: ingestion of contaminated food and water—commonly associated with undercooked shellfish; shellfish filter feed and therefore concentrate *V. cholera*
Skin and soft tissue infections: contact with contaminated water—commonly associated with recreational activity
High risk: immunocompromised, chronic liver disease, alcoholics

DIAGNOSIS
Culture: growth on selective agar—thiosulfate-citrate-bile-sucrose (TCBS) agar (differential agar for sucrose fermentation)
V. parahaemolyticus—blue-green colonies—sucrose non-fermenter
V. vulnificus—yellow or blue-green—sucrose fermentation is variable
See also ● 73, *Vibrio cholerae* ●
Oxidase positive

TREATMENT
GI infections: supportive
Ceftazidime, doxycycline

Explanation: Noncholera *Vibrio* may cause wound infections after contact with contaminated water. Similar to *V. cholerae,* these pathogens are also halotolerant and are associated with marine or estuarine environments. The organism most likely gains entry after a breach in the intact skin. Gastrointestinal infections may also occur after ingestion of contaminated food and water, and infections are commonly associated with shellfish, such as oysters. *Vibrio* species are curved gram-negative rods.

Micro gem: The cholera toxin increases cAMP. Other pathogens that also produce toxins that also increase cAMP include ● 68, Enterotoxigenic *Escherichia coli* (ETEC) ●, ● 61, *Bacillus cereus* ●, ● 109, *Bacillus anthracis* ●, and ● 23, *Bordetella pertussis* ●.

Vignette: A 40-year-old man presents with severe watery diarrhea of 3 days' duration. He had returned 4 days prior from a tour of several countries in Asia. He denies bloody stools but reports mucus in his stool. His temperature is 37.2°C (99.0°F). Upon examination, the man seems lethargic, his eyes are sunken, his skin feels cold and clammy, and his skin turgor is poor. The stool culture grows and organism on TCBS agar, and Gram stain shows curved gram-negative rods.

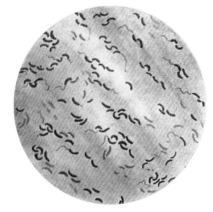

(1) *Source:* CDC public health library PHIL (phil.cdc.gov)
image No. 5324
(http://phil.cdc.gov/phil/details_linked.asp?pid=5324)

DESCRIPTION

Gram-negative rods (1), curved or comma-shaped

Many serogroups based on O antigen differences; two serogroups responsible for epidemics—O1 and O139

O1: predominant serogroup
   O1 serotypes: Inaba and Ogawa
   O1 biotypes: El tor and classical

INFECTIONS
PRIMARY

Gastrointestinal: cholera (enteritis) watery diarrhea—stools resemble rice water; may lead to dehydration

PATHOGENESIS

Flagella

Enterotoxin: cholera toxin—ADP-ribosylates G_s protein, stimulates adenylate cyclase and increases cAMP; results in fluid and electrolyte secretion and severe watery diarrhea

EPIDEMIOLOGY

Halotolerant

Transmission: contaminated food and water—commonly associated with undercooked shellfish; shellfish filter feed and therefore concentrate *V. cholerae*

Geographic distribution: endemic in Southeast Asia, India and Haiti

DIAGNOSIS

Culture: growth on selective agar—thiosulfate-citrate-bile-sucrose (TCBS) agar (differential agar for sucrose fermentation)
   Produces yellow colonies—sucrose fermenter
See also ● 72, Noncholera *Vibrio* ●
Oxidase positive

PREVENTION

Vaxchora (approved for used in the U.S. June 2016)—live, attenuated vaccine that targets serogroup O1

TREATMENT

Rehydration
Severe cases: azithromycin, doxycycline

ANIMATION

http://go.thieme.com/microb/Video73.1

Explanation: This man most likely has cholera caused by *Vibrio cholerae*, a curved gram-negative rod. This organism produces the cholera toxin, which increases cAMP and causes massive loss of electrolytes and water. This in turn leads to dehydration. Stools from infected patients are often referred to as "rice water" stool because of the profuse watery stools with flecks of mucus. This organism does not grow on "traditional" enteric media, and clinicians must notify the microbiologist if this organism is suspected. The selective media that is used to isolate this organism is TCBS agar.

Vignette: A 6-year-old girl presents with a 2-day history of abdominal pain, fever, vomiting, and bloody diarrhea. Her temperature is 38.7°C (101.7°F). Abdominal exam reveals tenderness of the right lower quadrant and rebound with guarding. CT scan rules out appendicitis. A CBC demonstrates elevated peripheral WBCs. The stool culture grows gram-negative rods on selective media.

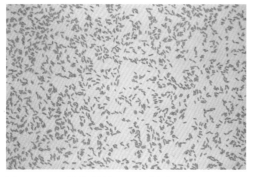

(1) *Source:* CDC public health library PHIL (phil.cdc.gov) image No. 2153 (http://phil.cdc.gov/phil/details_linked.asp?pid=2153)

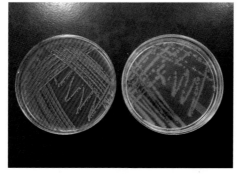

(2) MacConkey agar. Left side. lactose positive. Right side, lactose negative.

DESCRIPTION Gram-negative rods (1); part of *Enterobacteriaceae* family

See also ●129, *Klebsiella granulomatis* ●; ●131, *Klebsiella pneumoniae* ●; ●97, *Proteus* ●; ●47, *Salmonella enterica* serotype typhi and paratyphi ●; ●70, Nontyphoidal *Salmonella* ●; ●71, *Shigella* ●; ●138, *Yersinia pestis* ●

INFECTIONS

PRIMARY Gastrointestinal: colitis—watery or bloody diarrhea, fever may be present; pharyngitis may be present; children—mesenteric lymphadenitis; may mimic appendicitis

OTHER Post-infectious sequelae: erythema nodosum, reactive arthritis

PATHOGENESIS Adheres to and invades M cells in Peyer's patches of the terminal ileum; induces inflammation

EPIDEMIOLOGY Transmission:
Foodborne—commonly associated with undercooked pork
Ingestion of contaminated water
Contact with contaminated animals (rare)
High risk: individuals with hemochromatosis (because organism is siderophilic)

DIAGNOSIS Culture: lactose negative (2), *Y. enterocolitica* motile at 25°C and grows on selective media (Cefsulodin-Irgasan-Novobiocin Agar (CIN))
PCR from stool

TREATMENT Supportive
Severe cases: ceftriaxone plus aminoglycoside

ANIMATION http://go.thieme.com/microb/Video74.1

Explanation: *Yersina entercolitica*, a gram-negative rod, invades M cells in Peyer's patches of terminal, which leads to mesenteric lymphadenitis or pseudoappendicitis. Due to the propensity of the pathogen to infect lymphoid tissue, individuals may also present with sore throat/tonsillitis in addition to gastrointestinal symptoms. The organism is transmitted via contaminated food and is often associated with chitterlings. *Y. enterocolitica* and *pseudotuberculosis* grow on selective media and grow well at 25°C (room temperature) and at 4°C.

Vignette: A 21-year-old man presents with a 48-hour history of diarrhea and vomiting. He reports he feels more tired than usual and has a severe headache. At the time of examination his temperature is 38.9°C (102.0°F). Three days prior to the onset of symptoms, he returned from a spring-break vacation cruise. Within 72 hours of the onset of the symptoms, the symptoms subsided and he felt well again.

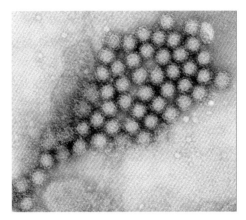

(1) *Source:* CDC/Charles D. Humphrey, PhD
    CDC public health library PHIL (phil.cdc.gov) image No. 10706
    (http://phil.cdc.gov/phil/details_linked.asp?pid=10706)

DESCRIPTION
Taxonomy: Calicivirus family; *Norovirus* genus
Virus properties: single-stranded, positive-sense RNA, non-enveloped (1)

INFECTIONS
 PRIMARY
Gastrointestinal: enteritis—watery diarrhea and vomiting; fever may be present

PATHOGENESIS
Blunting of villi of proximal small intestine

EPIDEMIOLOGY
Transmission:
  Foodborne—commonly associated foods include shellfish
  Person-to-person via fecal-oral route or vomitus (airborne droplets)
  Fomites
High risk: outbreaks often seen in group-related or close quarter settings (e.g., cruise ships)

DIAGNOSIS
Usually made on clinical findings
PCR from stool

TREATMENT
Supportive

Explanation: Norwalk virus is a single-stranded, positive-sense RNA virus that is part of the Calicivirus family. This virus causes a self-limiting gastroenteritis and is transmitted via contaminated food or water, or person to person from an infected individual. It is notable for causing outbreaks especially on cruise ships, college campuses, or in other close-quarter populations.

Micro gem: Rotavirus is the most common agent of diarrhea in children <2 years old.

Vignette: A 7-month-old girl presents to the emergency department in January with vomiting, fever, and watery diarrhea of 2 days' duration. Her father reports that although the baby has had more bowel movements than normal, she has had fewer wet diapers. The infant's temperature is 39.4°C (102.9°F). Upon examination, the infant's eyes and fontanelles are slightly sunken; she appears restless, and her mucous membranes are dry. Rotavirus antigen is detected by immunoassay.

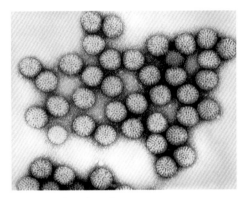

(1) *Source:* CDC/Dr. Erskine Palmer
   CDC public health library PHIL (phil.cdc.gov) image No. 178
   (http://phil.cdc.gov/phil/details_linked.asp?pid=178)

76 Rotavirus

DESCRIPTION

Taxonomy: Reovirus family. *See also* ●49, Colorado tick virus ●
Virus properties: double-stranded RNA, segmented genome, non-enveloped, double-layered capsid (1)

INFECTIONS
 PRIMARY

Gastrointestinal: enteritis—watery diarrhea and vomiting with fever; may lead to dehydration

PATHOGENESIS

Capsid protein NSP4 has cholera toxin-like activity
Transient malabsorption fats and carbohydrates
Blunting of villi

EPIDEMIOLOGY

Transmission: fecal-oral, fomites
Most common agent of diarrhea in children < 2 years old
Adults are often asymptomatic or have mild infections
Immunocompromised patients may have severe infection
Peaks in winter

DIAGNOSIS

Serology: antigen testing
PCR from stool

PREVENTION

Vaccine: Rotarix—live, attenuated vaccine; RotaTeq—live, reassortant vaccine

TREATMENT

Supportive

Explanation: Rotavirus is a double-stranded RNA virus. Although it may cause disease in adults, it is primarily an agent of gastroenteritis in young children, especially during the winter. Infections may lead to severe dehydration.

Micro gem: *Microsporidia,* ● 80, *Cryptosporidium* ●, and ● 81, *Cyclospora cayetanensis* ● are common nonbacterial agents of diarrhea in individuals with AIDS.

Vignette: A 53-year-old HIV-positive man presents with a 4-week history of diarrhea, abdominal pain, and weight loss. He denies blood in his stools. He has lost 15 pounds over the past month. His vitals are normal, but his abdominal exam reveals diffuse abdominal tenderness. His CD4 count is 69 cells/mm^3. Examination of his stool with a modified trichrome stain reveals oval spores.

(1)

DESCRIPTION
Fungi—previously classified as protozoa
Small, oval-shaped spores (1)
Commonly referred to as Microsporidia

INFECTIONS
PRIMARY
Gastrointestinal: diarrhea
    Immunocompetent—self-limiting
    Immunocompromised—chronic diarrhea and wasting
    May lead to biliary involvement

EPIDEMIOLOGY
Transmission: unclear (spores may be inhaled, ingested and can be found in contaminated food and water)
High risk: immunocompromised, especially individuals with AIDS with CD4 T-cells < 100 cells/mm^3 (2)

DIAGNOSIS
Microscopy: identification of spores from stool stained with modified trichrome sstain
PCR

TREATMENT
Albendazole

Explanation: Microsporidia were previously categorized as protozoa, but they are fungal organisms that form spores. There are many species of Microsporidia, including those in the *Enterocytozoon* and *Encephalitozoon* genera. In immunocompetent individuals, infections are often asymptomatic or self-limiting. However, immunocompromised individuals, especially AIDS patients, can present with serious chronic diarrhea. To visualize the oval spores of this pathogen, specimens are stained with the modified trichrome stain.

Vignette: A 6-year-old boy from rural Mississippi presents with lethargy. His mother says that he does not want to play and instead wants to sleep all the time. She also reports that he seems pale. On examination, his temperature is normal but his heart rate is elevated. Pallor is evident in his nail beds and conjunctivae. A CBC shows decreased hemoglobin and elevated eosinophils. A stool O&P demonstrates the presence of a thin-shelled, oval-shaped ovum.

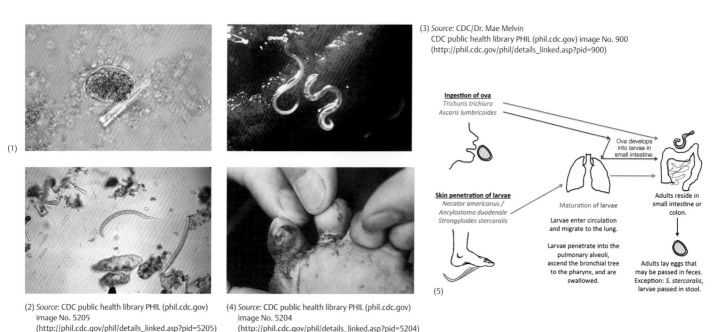

(1)

(2) *Source:* CDC public health library PHIL (phil.cdc.gov)
image No. 5205
(http://phil.cdc.gov/phil/details_linked.asp?pid=5205)

(4) *Source:* CDC public health library PHIL (phil.cdc.gov)
image No. 5204
(http://phil.cdc.gov/phil/details_linked.asp?pid=5204)

(3) *Source:* CDC/Dr. Mae Melvin
CDC public health library PHIL (phil.cdc.gov) image No. 900
(http://phil.cdc.gov/phil/details_linked.asp?pid=900)

Ingestion of ova
Trichuris trichiura
Ascaris lumbricoides

Ova develops into larvae in small intestine.

Adults reside in small intestine or colon.

Skin penetration of larvae
Necator americanus /
Ancylostoma duodenale
Strongyloides stercoralis

Maturation of larvae

Larvae enter circulation and migrate to the lung.

Larvae penetrate into the pulmonary alveoli, ascend the bronchial tree to the pharynx, and are swallowed.

Adults lay eggs that may be passed in feces. Exception: *S. stercoralis*, larvae passed in stool.

(5)

DESCRIPTION Nemathelminth / roundworm
Clinically important morphological forms: ova (eggs) (1), larvae (2), adult worms (3)
Commonly called hookworm

INFECTIONS

PRIMARY Skin and soft tissue: pruritus and maculopapular rash at site of entry (4)
Respiratory: asymptomatic or irritation of upper respiratory tract
Gastrointestinal: diarrhea, nausea, vomiting, abdominal pain

OTHER Complications: chronic nutritional impairment, anemia

LIFE CYCLE Eggs (1) passed in stool; eggs hatch in soil and develop into larvae (2); larvae penetrate human skin (*Ancylostoma*—ingestion as well); larvae migrate to lungs and are swallowed; develop into adults (3) in small intestine; adults lay eggs; eggs passed in stool (5)

EPIDEMIOLOGY Transmission: skin penetration of larva; *Ancylostoma*—also transmitted fecal-oral route (ingestion of ova)
Geographic distribution: endemic in sub-Saharan Africa, Asia, Latin America, and Caribbean; in the U.S., infections are more common in the South

DIAGNOSIS Microscopy: identification of ova from stool (1)
CBC: eosinophilia

TREATMENT Albendazole, mebendazole

Explanation: This boy has a hookworm infection, which is caused by *Necator americanus* or *Ancylostoma duodenale*. The larval form of the organism penetrates the skin of the host, initiating infection. Many infections are asymptomatic. However, if manifestations are present, symptoms will depend on where the worm is located in the body during that time. Cutaneous, pulmonary, or GI symptoms may be present. One of the main complications of infections is anemia, as presented in this case. Additionally, eosinophils are often elevated in helminthic infections, as seen here.

Vignette: A 4-year-old girl from rural Louisiana presents with a 3-day history of abdominal pain and vomiting. Her mother reports that the girl has not had a bowel movement in a few days. The child's vital signs are normal. On examination, her abdomen is tender and distended. Radiograph of the abdomen reveals obstruction and a "whirlpool pattern" with intraluminal worms.

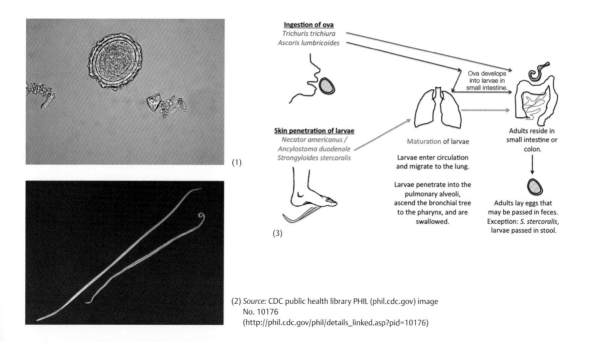

(1)

Ingestion of ova
Trichuris trichiura
Ascaris lumbricoides

Ova develops into larvae in small intestine.

Adults reside in small intestine or colon.

Skin penetration of larvae
Necator americanus /
Ancylostoma duodenale
Strongyloides stercoralis

Maturation of larvae

Larvae enter circulation and migrate to the lung.

Larvae penetrate into the pulmonary alveoli, ascend the bronchial tree to the pharynx, and are swallowed.

(3)

Adults lay eggs that may be passed in feces.
Exception: *S. stercoralis*, larvae passed in stool.

(2) *Source:* CDC public health library PHIL (phil.cdc.gov) image
No. 10176
(http://phil.cdc.gov/phil/details_linked.asp?pid=10176)

DESCRIPTION
Nemathelminth / roundworms
Clinically significant morphological forms: ova (eggs) (1), adult worms (2)

INFECTIONS

PRIMARY
Gastrointestinal: abdominal discomfort, diarrhea, nausea, anorexia
Respiratory: pneumonitis, hypersensitivity/urticaria

OTHER
Complications:
Malnutrition
Gastrointestinal: intestinal obstruction
Other: hepatobiliary and pancreas—cholecystitis, acute cholangitis, acute pancreatitis, and hepatic abscess (due to migration of parasite to biliary tree)

LIFE CYCLE
Eggs passed in stool, hatch into larvae in small intestine; larvae migrate to lungs and mature; swallowed; in small intestine mature into adults; adults lay eggs; eggs passed in the stool (3)

EPIDEMIOLOGY
Transmission: ingestion of ova from contaminated food and water
Geographic distribution: mainly in tropical climates; in the U.S., more common in the South
Co-infections with ● 88, *Trichiura trichuris* ● are common

DIAGNOSIS
Microscopy: identification of ova (1) or adult worms from stool or respiratory specimens (2)
Serology: antibody testing
CBC: eosinophilia

TREATMENT
Albendazole

Explanation: In the United States, helminthic infections are most often seen in the South. *Ascaris lumbricoides* is a roundworm that is transmitted via the fecal-oral route through contaminated food and water. Most infections are asymptomatic, but they can also result in mild gastrointestinal symptoms or respiratory symptoms as the worm migrates through the lungs. Complications of infection include intestinal obstruction. Radiographs may show a whirlpool like pattern as the mass of worms contrast against the gas.

Vignette: A 20-year-old college student visits the campus clinic with watery diarrhea of 3 days' duration. He states that he is nauseous and also complains of severe abdominal pain and fatigue. Upon examination, his temperature is 37.5°C (99.5°F). He has no rebound tenderness or guarding on palpitation of the abdomen. A modified acid-fast stain from the stool demonstrates the presence of an oocyst. The clinic physician notices that within 2 days of seeing this patient, 10 other students also present with similar findings.

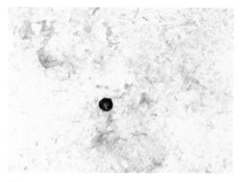

(1)

DESCRIPTION

Protozoa: apicomplexa—coccidia
Clinically significant morphological forms: oocyst
Clinically significant species: *C. parvum, C. hominis*

INFECTIONS
PRIMARY

Immunocompetent: often asymptomatic
Gastrointestinal: immunocompetent—mild watery diarrhea; immunocompromised/young children—severe watery diarrhea
Complication in immunocompromised: biliary disease

EPIDEMIOLOGY

Transmission: contaminated food and water (ingestion of oocyst)—commonly associated foods include raw produce
Associated with drinking water and fresh recreational water
High risk: immunocompromised, especially individuals with AIDS with CD4 T-cells < 100 cells/mm³ (1)

DIAGNOSIS

Microscopy: identification of oocyst from stool with modified acid-fast stain
PCR from stool

TREATMENT

Immunocompetent: nitazoxanide

Explanation: *Cryptosporidium* is a protozoan parasite that may contaminate drinking water. Infections with this pathogen are often asymptomatic, but acute infections may present with watery diarrhea, abdominal pain, and low-grade fever. The oocyst form of the parasite can be visualized microscopically with a modified acid-fast stain.

81 *Cyclospora cayetanensis*

Micro gem: *Cyclospora* and 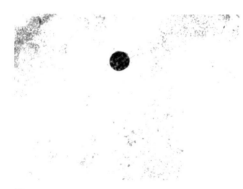 80, *Cryptosporidium* ● look very similar microscopically. Both pathogens stain with the modified acid-fast stain. The key difference is *Cyclospora* is larger than *Cryptosporidium* and *Cyclospora* is autofluorescent, which *Cryptosporidium* is not.

Vignette: A 57-year-old HIV-positive man presents with a 3-week history of diarrhea. He denies the presence of blood in his stool. He also complains of weight loss and being tired all the time. He has not traveled outside of the United States in several years. On exam, his vital signs are normal, but skin pallor is evident. Stool O&P results are negative, but a round oocyst is seen in a modified acid-fast smear. When viewed with a fluorescent microscope, the organism autofluoresces.

(1)

DESCRIPTION

Protozoa: apicomplexa—coccidia
Clinically significant morphological form: oocyst (1)

INFECTIONS
 PRIMARY

Gastrointestinal: watery diarrhea; may be chronic in HIV patients
   Complication in immunocompromised: biliary disease

EPIDEMIOLOGY

Waterborne pathogen
Transmission: ingestion of oocyst in contaminated food and water
   In U.S. mainly associated with contaminated water
   Not usually transmitted person to person
High risk for severe disease: young children, elderly, and immunocompromised, especially individuals with AIDS with CD4 T-cells < 100 cells/mm³ (2)

DIAGNOSIS

Microscopy: identification of oocyst from stool with modified acid-fast stain
Fluorescent microscopy: organism is autofluorescent
PCR from stool

TREATMENT

Trimethoprim-sulfamethoxazole

Explanation: *Cryptosporidium* and *Cyclospora* are both coccidian parasites that may cause chronic diarrhea in immunocompromised individuals. *Cyclospora* is most often transmitted via contaminated water. Both *Cyclospora* and *Cryptosporidium* stain with the modified acid-fast stain. However, *Cyclospora* is larger than *Cryptosporidium* and is autofluorescent, while *Cryptosporidium* is not. Hence, this man is more likely to have an infection with *Cyclospora*.

Vignette: A 33-year-old man presents to his primary care physician because he is tired all the time. He is an avid fisherman and spends much of his time in his cottage along Lake Michigan. He reports that he often consumes the fish that he catches. His vital signs are normal, and on exam skin pallor is evident. A CBC shows a hemoglobin level of 7.8 g/dL and a MCV of 120 fL. His LDH is slightly elevated and his serum vitamin B12 is significantly low.

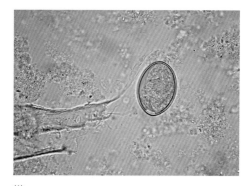

(1)

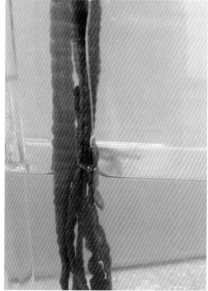

(2)

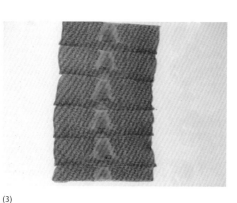

(3)

DESCRIPTION
Platyhelminth / flatworm: cestode / tapeworm
Clinically significant morphological forms: ova (eggs) (1), larvae, adult worms (2), with proglottids (3)
Alternative name: fish tapeworm

INFECTIONS
PRIMARY
Mainly asymptomatic
Gastrointestinal: diarrhea
　　Complication: megaloblastic anemia due to vitamin B12 deficiency

EPIDEMIOLOGY
Transmission: ingestion of larvae in undercooked freshwater fish
Associated with freshwater fish

DIAGNOSIS
Microscopy: microscopic identification of ova (1) or proglottids (3) from stool

TREATMENT
Praziquantel

Explanation: Infections with the tapeworm *Diphyllobothrium latum* are often asymptomatic. Mild gastrointestinal symptoms such as diarrhea and weight loss may occur, but often the major feature of infections with this pathogen is megaloblastic anemia, as in this case. This is one of the longest tapeworms of humans, and adult worms may reach up to 12 meters. There are several larval forms of the organism, and one of the larval forms lives in freshwater fish. Humans are infected after consumption of undercooked fish.

Micro gem: *Entamoeba histolytica* is considered the only clinically significant enteric amoeba and the only enteric amoeba in which antimicrobial treatment is indicated.

Vignette: A 56-year-old woman presents with diarrhea and fever of 4 days' duration. She reports that she saw blood and mucus in her stool, and she feels as though she constantly has to have a bowel movement. About 2 weeks ago she returned from Mexico. Her temperature is 38.2°C (100.8°F). Physical exam reveals mild abdominal tenderness. Her stool culture is reported as normal enteric flora. The stool O&P demonstrates the presence of a trophozoite with ingested red blood cells.

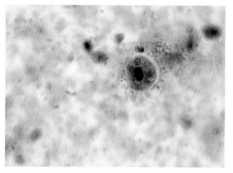 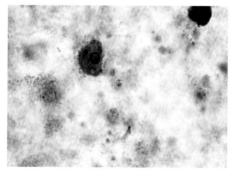 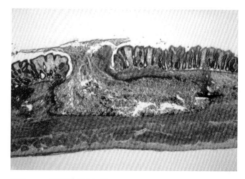

(1)

(2)

(3) Source: CDC/Dr. Melvin Mae
CDC public health library PHIL (phil.cdc.gov) image No. 416
(http://phil.cdc.gov/phil/details_linked.asp?pid=416)

DESCRIPTION

Protozoa: amoeba
Clinically significant morphological forms: cysts (1), trophozoites (2)

INFECTIONS

PRIMARY

Gastrointestinal: asymptomatic, watery diarrhea, amebic dysentery; mucosal ulcers [flask shaped (3)]

OTHER

Dissemination from GI tract
Liver: abscess
Nervous: abscess

EPIDEMIOLOGY

Transmission: ingestion of cysts in contaminated food or water
Geographic distribution: found worldwide; higher incidence in resource limited countries
High risk: travelers to endemic countries, men who have sex with men

DIAGNOSIS

Microscopy: identification of cysts or trophozoites from stool
PCR from stool

TREATMENT

GI infection: metronidazole

Explanation: *Entamoeba histolytica* is a protozoan parasite, and infections are most often asymptomatic. Manifestations, if present, include mild watery diarrhea or dysentery with blood and pus in the stool, tenesmus, and fever. This pathogen is more common in resource-limited regions of the world. One of the characteristic features of this pathogen that aids in diagnosis is the presence of ingested red blood cells within the trophozoite.

Vignette: A 3-year-old boy presents to the pediatrician with nausea and vomiting of 4 days' duration. His mother states that he has not been sleeping well at night and has been scratching his perianal area. A scotch-tape preparation from the perianal region is obtained and small, contact-lens–shaped ova are seen.

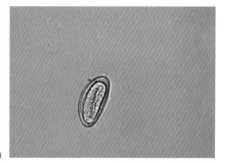
(1)

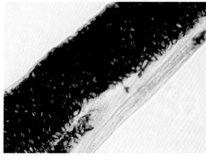
(2)

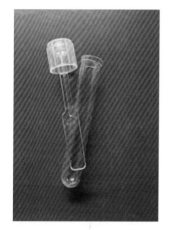
(3) Gravid female adult worm

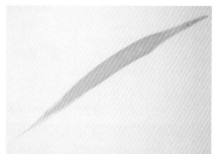
(4)

DESCRIPTION

Nemathelminth / roundworm
Clinically significant morphological forms: ova (eggs) (1), adult worms (2,3)
Alternative name: pinworm

INFECTIONS
 PRIMARY

Gastrointestinal: perianal pruitis, difficulty sleeping at night—because adult worms migrate to rectum at night and lay eggs

EPIDEMIOLOGY

Transmission:
 Ingestion of ova
 Person-to-person via fecal-oral route
 Fomites
 Self-infection—ova may get trapped in fingernails during anal itching and may then be ingested, leading to re-infection
High risk: young children

DIAGNOSIS

Microscopy: scotch-tape test or pinworm paddle (4) for identification of ova (1) or adult worms (2,3)

TREATMENT

Pyrantel pamoate, albendazole, mebendazole

Explanation: *Enterobius vermicularis* is a parasite that is commonly known as pinworm because adult worms are tiny, like a pinhead. Infection begins with ingestion of the eggs, also called ova, which hatch into larvae and mature into adults in the intestines. The females migrate to the perianal region, often at night, leading to perianal itching that is worse in the nighttime and causes difficulty sleeping. A scotch-tape preparation or a "pinworm paddle," which is paddle-shaped stick with a sticky surface, can be utilized to recover eggs and sometimes even a female adult worm. These worms are found worldwide and affect all age groups, but young children are particularly prone to infections with this pathogen.

Vignette: A 26-year-old man presents to his primary care physician with abdominal cramps and diarrhea of 1-week duration. He states he has been feeling more tired than normal, feels bloated, and is passing an unusual amount of gas. He mentions that he went camping about 2 weeks ago. At the time of the examination, his temperature is 37.1°C (98.8°F). A stool culture was negative for bacterial pathogens, but a trichrome stain from his stool demonstrates the presence of a pear-shaped trophozoite.

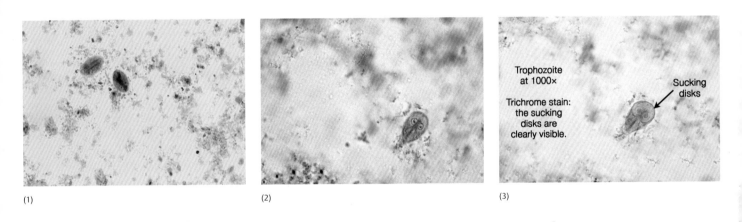

(1)　　　　　　　(2)　　　　　　　(3)

DESCRIPTION

Protozoa: flagellate
Clinically significant morphological forms: cysts (1), trophozoites (2,3)
Alternative names: *Giardia intestinalis* and *Giardia duodenalis*

INFECTIONS
 PRIMARY

Gastrointestinal: giardiasis—asymptomatic or foul-smelling watery diarrhea, flatulence, steatorrhea; complication—malabsorption

PATHOGENESIS

Trophozoite attaches to enterocyte brush border in duodenum with sucking disks, resulting in villous atrophy

EPIDEMIOLOGY

Transmission: infective form is cyst
 Contaminated food and water
 Person-to-person via fecal-oral route or sexual (anal-oral) contact
Associated with fresh water
High risk:
 Campers
 Young children
 Men who have sex with men
 Immunocompromised

DIAGNOSIS

Microscopy: identification of cyst (1) or trophozoites (2,3) from stool or duodenal aspirates
Serology: antigen testing
PCR from stool
Fecal fat test positive—indicative of steatorrhea

TREATMENT

Tinidazole, nitazoxanide, metronidazole

Explanation: This man's infection is most likely caused by *Giardia lamblia*, a parasite. The infectious cyst form of the organism is most often transmitted via ingestion of the pathogen, usually via contaminated water. In the intestines, the cyst develops into a trophozoite, with a flagella and an adhesive "sucking" disk that enables the organism to attach to the duodenal mucosa, although the organism does not invade the mucosa. Classic signs include diarrhea with foul-smelling stools, steatorrhea, and flatulence. Infected individuals may develop chronic infections with this organism that can lead to malabsorption.

Vignette: A 6-year-old girl presents with diarrhea, vomiting, and a stomachache of 3 days' duration. Both she and her mother deny blood in her stool. The mother reports the family returned from visiting relatives in Vietnam a few weeks ago. The girl's vital signs are normal. A CBC reveals eosinophilia. The stool culture is normal but the stool O&P demonstrates the presence of a *Strongyloides stercoralis* larva.

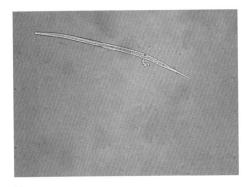

(1)

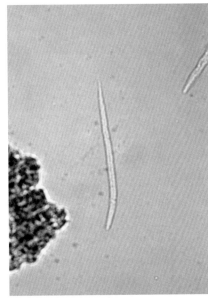

(2)

DESCRIPTION
Nemathelminth / roundworm
Clinically significant morphological forms: filariform (1) and rhabditiform (2) larvae

INFECTIONS
PRIMARY
Mainly asymptomatic
Gastrointestinal: diarrhea, abdominal pain
Respiratory: pneumonitis
Skin and soft tissue: urticaria

OTHER
Hyperinfection: increased parasite burden occurs due to auto-infection, and larvae may disseminate to any organ

LIFE CYCLE
Filariform larvae in soil: infects humans; migrates to lungs for further maturation; swallowed, and larvae develop into adult worms in small intestine; adults lay eggs and eggs develop into larvae; rhabditiform larvae passed in stool; rhabditiform larvae develop into filariform larvae in soil

EPIDEMIOLOGY
Transmission:
Skin penetration of filariform larva which can penetrate intact skin, such as bare feet
Autoinfection: rhabditiform larva develops into filariform larva in GI tract and life cycle can start again within the host
Geographic distribution: endemic in tropics and subtropics
Immunocompromised patients at are high risk for hyper-infection

DIAGNOSIS
Microscopy: identification of rhabditiform larvae from stool or respiratory specimens
Serology: antibody testing
Note: unlike ●79, *Ascaris lumbricoides* ● and ●78, *Ancylostoma duodenale* and *Necator americanus* ● infections, eosinophilia is often absent in strongyloidiasis

TREATMENT
Ivermectin

Explanation: Strongyloidiasis is caused by the helminthic parasite *Strongyloides stercoralis*. This pathogen is endemic in Southeast Asia and other tropical countries. Infections in the immunocompetent are often asymptomatic, and eosinophilia may be the only evidence of infection. The parasite can enter intact skin and migrates to lungs and then to the GI tract. Immunocompromised individuals may present with more serious hyperinfection or disseminated infections.

Vignette: A 48-year-old man presents with abdominal pain, vomiting, weight loss, and weakness. About 2 years ago, he had been diagnosed with chronic anemia and was subsequently treated. He has a history of eating raw beef. His vital signs and physical examination are unremarkable. Stool is collected for culture and O&P analysis. A round ovum with radial striations is isolated from the man's stool.

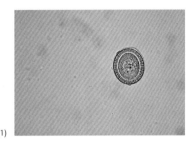

(1)

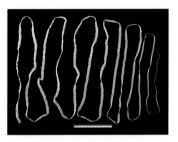

(2) *Source:* CDC public health library PHIL (phil.cdc.gov)
image No. 5260
(http://phil.cdc.gov/phil/details_linked.asp?pid=5260)

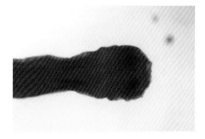

(3) *Source:* CDC/Dr. Mae Melvin
CDC public health library PHIL (phil.cdc.gov) image No. 10857
(http://phil.cdc.gov/phil/details_linked.asp?pid=10857)

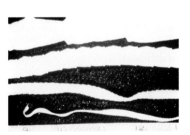

(4) *Source:* CDC public health library PHIL (phil.cdc.gov)
image No. 4833
(http://phil.cdc.gov/phil/details_linked.asp?pid=4833)

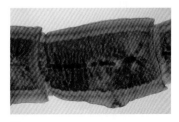

(5)

DESCRIPTION

Platyhelminth / flatworm: cestode / tapeworm
See also ● 13, *Taenia solium* ●
Clinically significant morphological forms: ova (eggs) (1), adult worms (2), with scolex (head) (3) and proglottids (section of body) (4,5)
Alternative name: beef tapeworm

INFECTIONS
PRIMARY

Gastrointestinal: asymptomatic or abdominal pain, nausea

EPIDEMIOLOGY

Transmission: foodborne (ingestion of cysticerci [larvae])—commonly associated food includes undercooked beef

DIAGNOSIS

Microscopy: identification of ova (1) or proglottids (4,5) from stool

TREATMENT

Praziquantel

Explanation: Infestation with the tapeworm *Taenia saginata* results in asymptomatic infections or nonspecific gastrointestinal symptoms, such as described in this case. The organism is transmitted via ingestion of undercooked beef. Proglottids (sections of the adult worm) or ova may be passed in the stool and assist with confirming the diagnosis.

Vignette: A 35-year-old woman presents with abdominal pain, intermittent diarrhea, and tenesmus of 3 weeks' duration. She had recently traveled to rural India. Her vital signs are normal, and the physical exam is unremarkable. A CBC reveals mild eosinophilia, and all other laboratory tests were normal. A stool O&P demonstrates the presence of football-shaped ova.

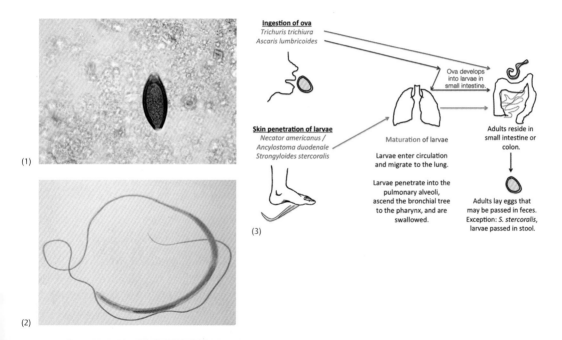

(1)

(2)

Ingestion of ova
Trichuris trichiura
Ascaris lumbricoides

Ova develops into larvae in small intestine.

Skin penetration of larvae
Necator americanus /
Ancylostoma duodenale
Strongyloides stercoralis

Maturation of larvae

Larvae enter circulation and migrate to the lung.

Larvae penetrate into the pulmonary alveoli, ascend the bronchial tree to the pharynx, and are swallowed.

(3)

Adults reside in small intestine or colon.

Adults lay eggs that may be passed in feces. Exception: *S. stercoralis*, larvae passed in stool.

DESCRIPTION
Nemathelminth / roundworm
Clinically significant morphological forms: ova (eggs) (1), adult worms (2)
Alternative name: whipworm

INFECTIONS
Mainly asymptomatic; symptoms mainly seen in heavy infections

PRIMARY
Gastrointestinal: diarrhea—may be bloody
Complication: rectal prolapse

LIFE CYCLE
Ova passed in stool and may be found in soil; ova ingested; ova in small intestine; develop into larvae; larvae develop into adult worms and reside in cecum and colon (3)

EPIDEMIOLOGY
Transmission: ingestion of ova in contaminated food and water
Geographic distribution: mainly in tropics and subtropics
High risk: children, individuals living in poor sanitary conditions
Co-infections with *Ascaris* are common

DIAGNOSIS
Microscopy: identification of ova from stool
Endoscopy to visualize adult worms
CBC: eosinophilia

TREATMENT
Mebendazole, albendazole

Explanation: Infections with the nematode *Trichuris trichiura* are most often asymptomatic or present with mild symptoms as this case. Other clinically significant intestinal nematodes include ● 78, *Ancylostoma duodenale* and *Necator americanus* ●, ● 86, *Strongyloides stercoralis* ●, and ● 79, *Ascaris lumbridoides* ●. Of these, only *Trichuris* adult worms reside in the cecum and colon (versus the small intestine). Infections are mainly seen in the tropics and subtropics, and are especially prevalent in Asia. Diagnosis is made by identification of the oval-shaped ova in stool or the adult worms via endoscopy. The ova contain two hyaline plugs at either pole, giving the ova a football-shaped appearance.

Micro gem: Hepatitis A and ● 93, Hepatitis E (HEV) ● viruses are transmitted by the fecal-oral route.

Vignette: A 48-year-old woman presents with fever, fatigue, dark yellow urine, and pale-colored stools of 6 days' duration. She has a lack of appetite and has felt nauseous for the past few days. She denies intravenous drug use, and has not engaged in sexual activity for the past 3 months. She returned from a 3-month Peace Corps mission to Laos approximately 6 weeks ago. Her temperature is 38.6°C (101.5°F), and physical examination reveals hepatosplenomegaly. ALT and AST are elevated and the hepatitis serology is positive for IgM anti-HAV.

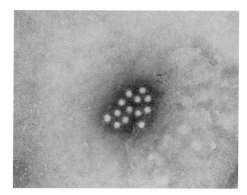

(1) *Source:* CDC/Dr. Herrmann
    CDC public health library PHIL (phil.cdc.gov) image No. 2739
    (http://phil.cdc.gov/phil/details_linked.asp?pid=2739)

89 Hepatitis A virus (HAV)

DESCRIPTION

Taxonomy: Picornavirus family; *Hepatovirus* genus
> *See also* ● 140, Non-polio Enterovirus ●; ● 8, Poliovirus ●; ● 33, Rhinovirus ●

Virus properties: single-stranded, positive-sense RNA, non-enveloped (1)

INFECTIONS

PRIMARY

Liver: acute hepatitis
> No chronic disease

EPIDEMIOLOGY

Transmission:
> Fecal-oral: often via contaminated food and water—commonly associated with shellfish and vegetables
> Sexual contact: oral-anal

Geographic distribution: found worldwide; but is endemic in Africa, Asia, Central and South America, Middle East, West Pacific

High risk:
> Travel to endemic area
> Poor sanitation
> Men who have sex with men
> Childcare workers
> Individuals living with someone infected with HAV
> HIV-positive individuals
> Illicit drug use

IgG against HAV provides life-long immunity from reinfection

DIAGNOSIS

Serology: antibody testing
> Acute: IgM anti–HAV
> Convalescence: IgG anti-HAV
> Past infection/immunity: total anti-HAV (IgM and IgG)

PREVENTION

Vaccine: inactivated vaccines (HAVRIX and VAQTA), combination HAV and HBV vaccine

TREATMENT

Supportive

Explanation: This woman most likely has acute hepatitis A. The hepatitis A virus belongs to the Picornavirus family, which also includes Enteroviruses, such as Coxsackie virus, Poliovirus, and Rhinovirus. Hepatitis A is transmitted fecal-orally. High-risk individuals include travelers to endemic regions, such as in this case. IgM anti-HAV is positive in acute infections. IgG anti-HAV peaks during the convalescent phase of infection and confers enduring protection.

Micro gem: Hepatitis B, ●91, Hepatitis C (HCV)●, and ●92, Hepatitis D (HDV)● viruses are agents of acute **and chronic** hepatitis.

Vignette: A 31-year-old man presents with a 1-week history of fever, abdominal pain, nausea, and vomiting. He was worried and sought medical attention when he noticed that his eyes turned yellow. He denies injection drug use, and has not traveled outside of the United States recently. He admits to recent sexual activity and has had several partners, both male and female, within the past 6 months. He is not up-to-date with vaccinations. His temperature is 38.6°C (101.5°F). On examination his sclera are icteric and hepatosplenomegaly is present. ALT is significantly elevated. His hepatitis serology panel is positive for HBsAg, total anti-HBc, and IgM anti-HBc, and negative for anti-HBs.

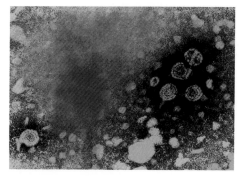

(1) *Source:* CDC/Dr. Erksine Palmer
   CDC public health library PHIL (phil.cdc.gov) image No. 10755
   (http://phil.cdc.gov/phil/details_linked.asp?pid=10755)

90 Hepatitis B virus (HBV)

DESCRIPTION
Taxonomy: Hepadnavirus family
Virus properties: partially double-stranded DNA, enveloped (1)
Encodes a reverse transcriptase

INFECTIONS
PRIMARY
Liver: acute and chronic hepatitis
Complications of chronic infections: cirrhosis, liver failure, increased risk of developing hepatocellular carcinoma

EPIDEMIOLOGY
Transmission:
Contact with infected body fluids such as blood and semen (i.e., needlestick, sexual)
Vertical (*in utero*, perinatal, postnatal)
Geographic distribution: found worldwide; endemic regions include parts of Africa, Pacific Islands, South East Asia, Central and Eastern Europe, Central and South America
High risk:
Travel to an endemic area
Injection drug use
Men who have sex with men
Healthcare workers
Infants born to HBV infected mother
Unprotected sex with multiple partners or an individual with HBV
Individuals living with someone infected with HBV

DIAGNOSIS
Serology: antibody testing (not a complete list of serological markers):
IgM anti–hepatitis B core (HBc): acute
Hepatitis B surface antigen (HBsAg): acute and chronic (> 6 months)
Total anti-HBc: acute, chronic, resolved
Anti-HBs: recovery/immunity
Hepatitis B envelope antigen (HBeAg): marker of infectivity
PCR for viral load/quantification
Genotype sequencing

PREVENTION
Vaccine: recombination vaccines (Engerix-B, Recombivax HB), combination HAV and HBV vaccine

TREATMENT
Will depend on HBeAg results, viral load, liver enzyme and level of fibrosis
Pegylated interferon alpha 2a, entecavir, tenofovir

Explanation: This patient has acute hepatitis B, caused by the DNA virus hepatitis B. This pathogen is transmitted percutaneously, permucosally, and vertically. In this case, the pathogen was most likely transmitted sexually. This patient is most likely not immunized against hepatitis B virus, as indicated by the negative anti-HBs. Chronic hepatitis B infections may develop and may lead to cirrhosis, liver failure, or hepatocellular carcinoma.

Micro gem: Infections with ● 90, Hepatitis B (HBV) ● and Hepatitis C viruses increase the risk of developing hepatocellular carcinoma.

Vignette: A 54-year-old man is in the emergency department following a motor vehicle accident. He claims he is fine and is not visibly hurt. His vitals and physical examination are unremarkable. A CBC and routine chemistry profile are ordered, and the CBC is normal, but the chemistry panel demonstrates significantly elevated AST and ALT. The man is discharged but is referred to a gastroenterologist.

A few weeks later the man visits the gastroenterologist. His history is significant for injection drug use, but he denies using illicit drugs for the past 20 years. His vital signs and physical examination are unremarkable. His hepatitis serology panel is positive for anti-HCV and HCV RNA.

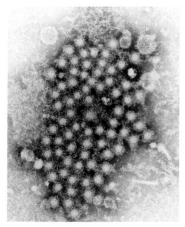

(1) *Source:* CDC/E.H. Cook, Jr.
   CDC public health library PHIL (phil.cdc.gov) image No. 8153
   (http://phil.cdc.gov/phil/details_linked.asp?pid=8153)

91 Hepatitis C virus (HCV)

DESCRIPTION
Taxonomy: Flavivirus family.
See also ● 7, Arthropod borne Flaviviruses ●
Virus properties: single-stranded, positive-sense RNA, enveloped (1)
6 genotypes—in the U.S., genotype 1 is the most common

INFECTIONS
PRIMARY
Liver: acute and chronic hepatitis (85% of individuals develop chronic disease)
    Complications of chronic infections: cirrhosis, increased risk of developing hepatocellular carcinoma

EPIDEMIOLOGY
Transmission:
    Primarily via contact with infected blood (contaminated needles, blood products)
    Less common—sexual contact, vertical (usually perinatal)
Geographic distribution: found worldwide; endemic in Central and East Asia, North Africa and, Middle East
High risk:
    Individuals who have been incarcerated
    Receipt of piercing or tattoo in unsanitary conditions
    Illicit drug use
    Men who have sex with men
    Healthcare workers
    Infants born to HCV infected mother
    Blood transfusion prior to 1999

DIAGNOSIS
Antibody testing: anti-HCV: present in current infection or past/resolved infection
    Note: cannot distinguish acute from chronic infection
PCR for viral load/quantification
Genotype sequencing

TREATMENT
Will depend on genotype, level of fibrosis, co-infections, previous HCV treatment, and other indicators
Recommended treatment regimens are fluid—consult American Association for the Study of Liver Disease and Infectious Disease Society of America's most recent recommendations
Classes of agents utilized in HCV therapy include:
    Interferons
    Protease inhibitors—inhibit the HCV protease, NS3/4A; example—grazoprevir
    NS5A inhibitors—NS5A is a nonstructural protein involved in viral replication and assembly; examples—elbasvir, ledipasvir
    Polymerase inhibitors—inhibit HSV RNA-depended-RNA-polymerase, NS5B; example—sofosbuvir
Example current treatment for genotype 1a—elbasvir plus grazoprevir OR ledipasvir plus sofosbuvir

Explanation: This man most likely has chronic hepatitis C. Hepatitis C is a RNA virus and infections may be acute or chronic. A significant proportion of individuals will develop chronic infections, which may then lead to liver failure, cirrhosis, or hepatocellular carcinoma. Infections are most often asymptomatic, but can also present with the typical symptoms of viral hepatitis. Hepatitis C is transmitted via contact with blood from an infected individual, and may occur via sharing of contaminated needles and contaminated blood products. Less common modes of transmission include sexual and vertical transmission.

Vignette: A 44-year-old woman presents with a 2-week history of abdominal pain, fever, nausea, and vomiting. She denies injection drug use, and has not traveled outside of the United States recently. On examination, she is icteric, and hepatosplenomegaly is evident. ALT and AST are elevated. Her hepatitis serology panel is positive for HBsAg, total anti-HBc, IgM anti-HBc, and anti-HDV, and is negative for anti-HBs.

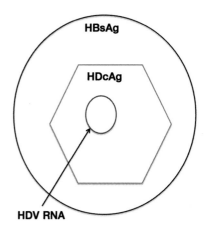

- The HDV core antigen (HDcAg) depends on the synthesis of the HBV surface antigen (HBsAg) to support replication and expression.
- Without HBsAg coating, HDV cannot survive, multiply, or infect on its own.

(1)

92 Hepatitis D virus (HDV)

DESCRIPTION

Requires ● 90, Hepatitis B virus (HBV) ● for replication

Virus properties: incomplete/defective virus particle—dependent on hepatitis B virus for replication and infection, single-stranded, negative-sense RNA (1)

INFECTIONS

PRIMARY

Liver: hepatitis

- Co-infection: infected with HDV at the same time as HBV
- Superinfection: chronic infection with HBV first, then infection with HDV

EPIDEMIOLOGY

Transmission: same as hepatitis B (infected blood and body fluids)

DIAGNOSIS

Antibody testing: anti-HDV IgM

TREATMENT

None recommended; see HBV

Explanation: This patient has a co-infection with HBV and HDV. HDV requires HBV for replication. Infections with HBV may occur at the same time, resulting in co-infection, as in this case, or individuals may have a chronic HBV infection and then contract HDV, resulting in superinfection.

Vignette: A 26-year-old man presents with a 1-week history of fever, vomiting and nausea, yellow urine, and pale-colored stools. He denies intravenous drug use. He currently has one female sexual partner. About 3 months ago he returned from a vacation to Belize. His temperature is 38.6°C (101.5°F), and physical examination reveals hepatomegaly. ALT and AST are elevated, and the hepatitis serology panel is positive for IgG anti-HAV, anti-HBs, and IgG anti-HEV.

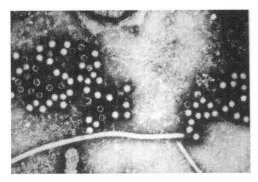

(1) *Source:* CDC public health library PHIL (phil.cdc.gov) image No. 5605
(http://phil.cdc.gov/phil/details_linked.asp?pid=5605)

93 Hepatitis E virus (HEV)

DESCRIPTION
Taxonomy: Hepevirus family
Virus properties: single-stranded, positive-sense RNA, non-enveloped (1)
Four genotypes

INFECTIONS
PRIMARY

Liver: acute hepatitis
No chronic disease

EPIDEMIOLOGY
Transmission: fecal-oral route—most often contaminated drinking water
Geographic distribution: not as common in the U.S. as other hepatitis viruses; endemic in Africa, Asia, Middle East and Central America
High risk:
Travel to an endemic region
Pregnant females, especially in third trimester, are at risk for more serious sequelae, including hepatic failure

DIAGNOSIS
Serology: antibody testing
IgM anti–HEV : acute infection
IgG anti-HEV: late acute phase and convalescence
PCR

TREATMENT
Supportive

Explanation: Hepatitis E virus is transmitted via contaminated water and is more common in resource-limited countries than in the United Sates. Hepatitis E is a single-stranded RNA virus, and infections have an average incubation of 40 days. During acute infections, liver enzymes are usually significantly elevated. The IgM anti-HEV is positive early on and disappears within 4 to 5 months. The IgG anti-HEV is positive shortly after the IgM and may be positive for life.

Micro gem: *Clonorchis sinensis* and ● 96, *Fasciola hepatica* ● are clinically significant flukes that may infect the liver.

Vignette: An otherwise healthy 55-year-old man complains of fatigue, indigestion, and intermittent abdominal pain and diarrhea of 4 weeks' duration. He denies blood in his stool. About 2 months ago he returned from a business trip to China. His vital signs are normal. Abdominal exam reveals tenderness in the right upper quadrant. Significant laboratory results include an elevated alkaline phosphatase. An endoscopic retrograde cholangiopancreatography (ERCP) shows the presence of several worms, approximately 10 mm in length, in the bile duct.

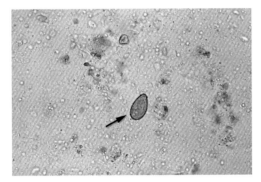

(1) *Source:* CDC public health library PHIL (phil.cdc.gov) image No. 5248
     (http://phil.cdc.gov/phil/details_linked.asp?pid=5248)

DESCRIPTION

Platyhelminth / flatworm: trematode / fluke
Clinically significant morphological forms: ova (1), larvae (several forms including cercariae and metacercariae)
Alternative name: liver fluke or Chinese liver fluke

INFECTIONS
PRIMARY

Mainly asymptomatic; infections may be acute or chronic
Gastrointestinal (usually acute): abdominal pain, flatulence, diarrhea, hepatomegaly may be present
Liver/biliary (usually chronic): weight loss, diarrhea, abdominal discomfort
Complications include obstructive jaundice, cholangitis, liver abscess, cholangiocarcinoma

LIFE CYCLE

Ova passed in stool: ingested by freshwater snail and develops into larva; snail ingested by freshwater fish; humans ingest fish; larva excysts in small intestine and develop into adult worms; adult worms live in biliary ducts

EPIDEMIOLOGY

Transmission: ingestion of undercooked freshwater fish
Geographic distribution: endemic in East Asia (Korea, China, Taiwan, Japan, Vietnam)

DIAGNOSIS

Microscopy: identification of ova (1) from stool or bile
CBC: eosinophilia
Elevated liver function tests

TREATMENT

Praziquantel

Explanation: Infections with the fluke *Clonorchis sinensis* may be acute or chronic. Acute infections may be asymptomatic or result in nonspecific findings and abdominal pain. Chronic infections occur as a result of the adult worms residing in the bile duct. An elevated alkaline phosphatase is consistent with biliary obstruction. Symptoms may include fatigue, dyspepsia, weight loss, and diarrhea. This fluke species is mainly seen in the Far East in countries such as China, and is associated with the intestine of raw or undercooked freshwater fish. Ova may be seen in the stool or bile, and adult worms may be seen with ERCP.

Vignette: A 35-year-old man, who recently immigrated from Iraq, presents with abdominal pain. He states he has had intermittent abdominal pain for approximately 5 years. During the past 3 years, the pain has been more constant. During the last 2 months the pain has become debilitating. He describes the pain as a dull pain that becomes sharp with inhalation. The right upper quadrant of his abdomen is soft and tender with palpation. There is pain with palpation of liver edge at the right costal margin. His physical exam is otherwise normal. Laboratory studies show elevated AST and ALT levels. A MRI of his abdomen shows a left hepatic lobe cystic mass.

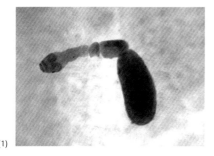

(1)

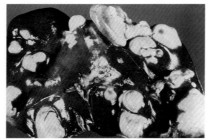

(2) *Source:* CDC/Dr. Peter Trenton Ruebrush
CDC public health library PHIL (phil.cdc.gov) image No. 14930
(http://phil.cdc.gov/phil/details_linked.asp?pid=14930)

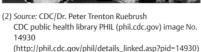

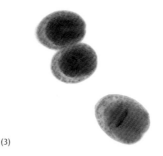

(3)

(5) *Source:* CDC/Dr. Kagen
CDC public health library PHIL (phil.cdc.gov) image No. 2865
(http://phil.cdc.gov/phil/details_linked.asp?pid=2865)

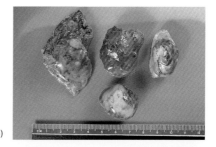

(4)

DESCRIPTION

Platyhelminth / flatworm: cestode / tapeworm
Clinically significant morphological forms: ova (eggs), onchospheres (larvae), adult worms (1) with scolex and proglottids
Hydatid sand consists of scolices, daughter cysts and hooks

INFECTIONS
PRIMARY

Initial infection: mainly asymptomatic
Liver (chronic infection): development hydatid cyst—fluid-filled cyst (2) with hydatid sand (3,4), which may result in abdominal pain, nausea and vomiting
    Complications: rupture of cyst in biliary tree resulting in cholangitis, pancreatitis and obstructive jaundice

OTHER

Respiratory: development of hydatid cyst in lungs (5)—may manifest as cough, hemoptysis and dyspnea
Rupture of the cyst may lead to anaphylaxis

EPIDEMIOLOGY

Dogs are the definite hosts and are infected with larvae after ingestion of viscera of sheep, goats, and pigs (intermediate hosts)
Transmission: humans infected after ingestion of food, water, or soil contaminated with infected dog feces
Geographic distribution: higher incidence in the Mediterranean, Middle East, sub-Saharan Africa, Russia and parts of China

DIAGNOSIS

Serology: antibody testing
Imaging—presence of cyst-like lesion
Once diagnosis is confirmed, cyst may be removed—cyst fluid may contain hydatid sand

TREATMENT

Albendazole

ANIMATION

http://go.thieme.com/microb/Video95.1

Explanation: This man is most likely to have hydatid liver cyst, caused by the tapeworm *Echinococcus granulosus*. Humans are most often infected following ingestion of food or water contaminated with feces from an infected animal. Infections are more common in countries of the Middle East, including Iraq. Initial infections are usually asymptomatic. As the cyst grows, individuals become asymptomatic. These fluid-filled cysts are usually in the liver or lungs. The fluid contains hydatid sand, which contains daughter cysts, scolices, and hooks of the worm. The cyst should not be removed until the diagnosis is confirmed, with imaging and serology.

Vignette: A 20-year-old woman visits the campus clinic complaining of a stomachache and fever of 1-week duration. She reports she has not had an appetite for several weeks and has lost almost 10 pounds. History reveals that she returned from a semester abroad in Peru about 1 month ago. She reports that in Peru she always drank bottled or filtered water and denies eating from street vendors. She does remember consuming edible flowers that were given to her by her host family. On exam her temperature is 38.4°C (101.1°F). Abdominal exam reveals right upper quadrant tenderness and hepatomegaly. A stool specimen demonstrates several oval-shaped ova.

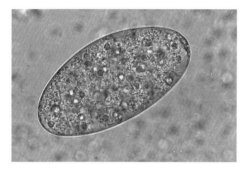

(1) *Source:* CDC/Dr. Mae Melvin
   CDC public health library PHIL (phil.cdc.gov) image No. 15219
   (http://phil.cdc.gov/phil/details_linked.asp?pid=15219)

DESCRIPTION   Platyhelminth / flatworm: trematode / fluke
Clinically significant morphological forms: ova (eggs) (1)
Alternative name: liver fluke

INFECTIONS
PRIMARY   Liver (acute): abdominal pain, jaundice, hepatosplenomegaly
Biliary (chronic): obstructive jaundice, cholangitis, choleithiasis

LIFE CYCLE   Ova passed in feces (humans and herbivores); ova in fresh water; form miracidia; invade snails; snails release larval form (cercariae); larvae (metacercariae) encyst on fresh water vegetation; humans ingest fresh water plants

EPIDEMIOLOGY   Transmission: ingestion of fresh water vegetation, such as watercress
Geographic distribution: found worldwide but endemic in Central and South America, Asia, Europe, Africa, and Middle East

DIAGNOSIS   Microscopy: identification of ova from stool or bile
CBC: eosinophilia

TREATMENT   Triclabendazole

Explanation: *Fasciola hepatica* is a flatworm that is endemic in several regions of the world, including countries in Central and South America, such as Peru and Bolivia. The pathogen is transmitted to humans via ingestion of contaminated water plants. The larva migrates from the small intestine to the liver and bile ducts, where adult worms reside. Infections may be acute or chronic, and symptoms are often nonspecific. The adults lay eggs (ova), and ova may be seen in the stool.

97 *Proteus mirabilis*

Micro gem: Two key characteristics of *Proteus mirabilis* is the production of urease and the ability of this pathogen to swarm on blood agar.

Vignette: A 38-year-old woman presents with urinary urgency and frequency of 3 days duration. That morning she noted what appeared to be blood in her urine and also had severe pain on her right side. Upon examination her temperature is 37.9°C (100.2°F), and she has costovertebral angle tenderness on the right side. She has no rebound tenderness or guarding on palpitation of her abdomen. Blood was collected for a CBC, which demonstrates a peripheral WBC count of 14.1×10^9/L. Urinalysis is positive for blood, protein, nitrites, and leukocyte esterase. An abdominal CT was ordered because of prior history of stones; the scan demonstrates three nonobstructing calculi, all less than 0.5 cm diameter, in the right collecting system.

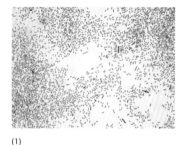

(1)

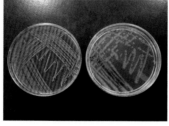

(2) MacConkey agar. Left, lactose positive. Right, lactose negative.

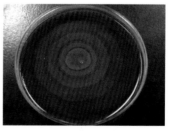

(3)

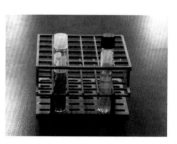

(4) Left, urease positive. Right, urease negative.

DESCRIPTION

Gram-negative rods (1); part of family *Enterobacteriaceae*
See also ● 129, *Escherichia coli* ●; ● 103, *Klebsiella granulo-matis* ●; ● 131, *Klebsiella pneumoniae* ●; ● 47, *Salmonella enterica* serotype typhi and paratyphi ●; ● 70, Nontyphoidal *Salmonella* ●; ● 71, *Shigella* ●; ● 74, *Yersinia enterocolitica* and *pseudotuberculosis* ●; ● 138, *Yersinia pestis* ●

INFECTIONS

PRIMARY

Renal/urinary: UTIs—renal calculi may be present

OTHER

Skin and soft tissue: wounds
Systemic: bacteremia

PATHOGENESIS

Fimbriae/pili: adherence to epithelium
Flagella
Urease: breaks down urea and produces ammonia

EPIDEMIOLOGY

Normal GI microbiota; may colonize skin and oral mucosa
Transmission: usually displacement of endogenous strains
UTIs associated with indwelling catheters or anatomic or functional abnormalities of the urinary tract
Common nosocomial pathogen

DIAGNOSIS

Culture: lactose negative (2), swarming colonies on blood agar (3)—due to motility by flagella, urease positive (4)
Urinalysis may demonstrate alkaline urine and struvite (triple phosphate) crystals due to urease production
PUNCH = Urease positive organisms
Proteus mirabilis; ● 104, **U**reaplasma ●; ● 28, **N**ocardia ●; ● 11, **C**ryptococcus neoformans and gatti ●; ● 69, **H**elicobacter pylori ●

TREATMENT

Depends on infection type
UTI and other non-life-threatening infections—trimethoprim-sulfamethoxazole, ciprofloxacin, amoxicillin-clavulanate
For more serious infections piperacillin-tazobactam

Explanation: This woman has pyelonephritis caused by *Proteus mirabilis*, a gram-negative rod. Due to the motility of this organism, swarming is often noted on blood agar. On MacConkey agar, which is selective for gram-negative rods and differential, *P. mirabilis* is clear due to lack of lactose fermentation. *Proteus* produces urease, which breaks down urea into carbon dioxide and ammonia and causes elevated urinary pH levels. Increases in urine pH can contribute to direct renal toxicity and to urinary stone formation. Urinary stones can result in further renal damage by obstructing urine flow. Often struvite crystals (also called triple phosphate) are observed in the urine of patients with UTIs caused by *Proteus*.

Micro gem: All staphylococci are catalase positive. Only ● 134, *Staphylococcus aureus* ● is coagulase positive. All other staphylococci are referred to as coagulase negative staphylococci, including *Staphylococcus saprophyticus*.

Vignette: A 25-year-old woman presents with a 3-day history of painful urination and increased frequency and urgency of urination. The woman recently returned from her honeymoon. A urinalysis demonstrates the presence of leukocyte esterase and is negative for nitrates. The urine culture grows > 100,000 CFUs of a gram-positive coccus in clusters. The organism is coagulase-negative and novobiocin resistant.

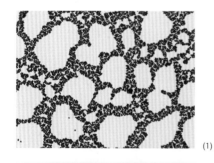

(1)

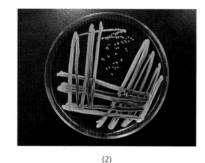

(2)

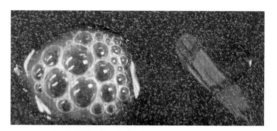

(3) Left, catalase positive.
Right, catalase negative.

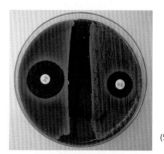

(5) Left, novobiocin sensitive.
Right, novobiocin resistant.

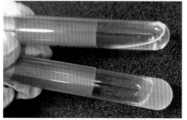

(4) Top, coagulase negative.
Bottom, coagulase positive.

DESCRIPTION
Gram-positive cocci in clusters (1)
A type of coagulase-negative staphylococci

INFECTIONS
PRIMARY
Renal/urinary: UTIs—often referred to as honeymoon cystitis due to its association with sexually active females

PATHOGENESIS
Mucosal adhesins
Urease—breaks down urea and produces ammonia

EPIDEMIOLOGY
Associated with young sexually active females

DIAGNOSIS
Culture (2): catalase-positive (3), coagulase-negative (4), novobiocin resistant (5)
Urinalysis may demonstrate alkaline urine and struvite (triple phosphate) crystals due to urease production

TREATMENT
Cephalexin, amoxicillin-clavulanate, trimethoprim-sulfamethoxazole

Explanation: *Staphylococcus saprophyticus* is a gram-positive coccus in clusters. Leukocyte esterase is an enzyme produced by WBCs and may indicate pyuria. Some bacteria, most notably gram-negative rods, convert nitrates to nitrites. Since the causative agent in this case is Gram positive, the nitrate is negative. *S. saprophyticus* is a coagulase-negative staphylococci and is novobiocin resistant. Infections with this organism are often referred to as "honeymoon cystitis."

Vignette: A 25-year-old man presents with a 3-month history of dull belly pain and periodic blood in his urine. He immigrated to the United States from Ghana approximately 1 year ago. He reports that he has been experiencing increased frequency of urination and slight pain when urinating. He is otherwise healthy, and his vital signs and physical examination are unremarkable. Abdominal ultrasound demonstrates thickening of the bladder wall, and a CT scan shows calcification of the bladder wall and ureter. A bladder biopsy reveals granulomas and inflammation.

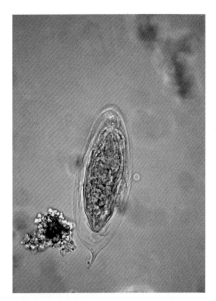

(1)

DESCRIPTION
Platyhelminth / flatworm: trematode / fluke
Clinically significant morphological forms: ova (eggs) (1)

INFECTIONS
PRIMARY
Renal/urinary: urinary schistosomiasis—hematuria, dysuria
Chronic infections may lead to granulomatous inflammation and are associated with bladder carcinoma

LIFE CYCLE
Ova released in fresh water from human urine; develop into miracidia; miracidia penetrate snails; miracidia mature to larvae in snails; snails release cercariae; cercariae penetrate human skin; enter circulation and migrate to hepatic portal system; mature into adults; adults migrate and live in venous plexus of bladder

EPIDEMIOLOGY
Transmission: contact with contaminated fresh water
Geographic distribution: mainly seen in sub-Saharan Africa and the Middle East

DIAGNOSIS
Microscopy: identification of ova in urine which are oval shaped with prominent terminal spine (1)
Serology: antibody testing
CBC: eosinophilia

TREATMENT
Praziquantel

Explanation: This patient has a chronic infection with the trematode (fluke) *Schistosoma haematobium*. *S. haematobium* is also referred to as the bladder fluke because the pathogen resides in the venous plexus of the bladder. Humans become infected with schistosomes after contact with freshwater contaminated with larvae which can penetrate the skin. In the human host, the larvae develop into adults that lay eggs, which are then passed in the urine.

See also ● 122, *Schistosoma mansoni* and *japonicum* ●

Micro gem: ●*Chlamydia trachomatis* ●, ● 105, *Neisseria gonorrhoeae* ●, and Herpes simplex virus-2 (● 139, Herpes simplex virus (HSV)-1 and -2 ●) are the most common agents of neonatal eye infections.

Vignette 1: A 5-day-old girl is brought to her pediatrician with a yellowish discharge from her eyes and swollen eyelids. Other than the conjunctivitis, the physical examination is unremarkable. A Gram stain from the discharge reveals no organisms. The pathogen grows in cell culture, and a Giemsa stain of the organism reveals intracellular inclusion bodies.

Vignette 2: A 21-year-old sexually active woman complains of vaginal discharge and abdominal and pelvic pain of 2 weeks' duration. She is afebrile and her physical exam demonstrates abdominal tenderness and mucopurulent cervical discharge. A cervical swab is obtained for Gram stain and culture and the Gram stain is reported as normal vaginal flora. After 2 days the culture is reported as normal vaginal flora, no *Neisseria gonorrhoeae* isolated.

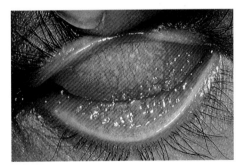
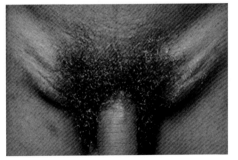
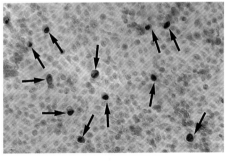

(1) *Source:* CDC/Susan Lindsley
CDC public health library PHIL (phil.cdc.gov) image No. 15193
(http://phil.cdc.gov/phil/details_linked.asp?pid=15193)

(2) *Source:*
Herbert L. Fred, MD and Hendrik A. van Dijk (http://cnx.org/content/m14883/latest/)
[CC BY-SA 2.0 (http://creativecommons.org/licenses/by-sa/2.0)], via Wikimedia Commons

(3) *Source:* CDC/ Dr. E. Arum, Dr. N. Jacobs
CDC public health library PHIL (phil.cdc.gov) image No. 6428
(http://phil.cdc.gov/phil/details_linked.asp?pid=6428)

100 *Chlamydia trachomatis*

DESCRIPTION

Rod-shaped
  Cell wall has LPS but lacks peptidoglycan
  Does not Gram stain
  Cannot synthesize its own ATP
Clinically significant serovars: A, B, Ba and C, D–K, L1, L2, L3
Obligate intracellular pathogen
  Host cell:
    A, B, Ba and C, D–K—epithelial cell
    L1–L3—macrophage
Morphological forms:
  Elementary body—infective, nonreplicating form
  Reticulate body—noninfectious, replicating form

INFECTIONS

PRIMARY

Post-natal:
Head and neck: eye
  Serovars A, B, Ba and C
    Trachoma—in-turned eyelids and eyelashes which may lead to scaring and blindness
  Serovars D–K
    Inclusion conjunctivitis in adults (1)
Reproductive:
  Serovars D–K
    Genital chlamydia: asymptomatic or symptomatic urethritis (nongonococcal) and cervicitis
    Complications: pelvic inflammatory disease (PID)—associated with Fitz-Hugh–Curtis syndrome

Serovars L1, L2, L3
  Lymphogranuloma venereum (LGV) (2)—painless papule with painful lymphadenopathy; positive groove sign
  See also ●102, *Haemophilus ducreyi* ●; ●103, *Klebsiella granulomatis* ●; ●106, *Treponema pallidum* ●; ●139, Herpes simplex virus (HSV)-1 and -2 ●
Neonatal: serovars D–K
  Head and neck: eye—conjunctivitis (ophthalmia neonatorum) —5 to 14 days after birth
  Respiratory: pneumonia

OTHER

Post-infectious sequelae
Musculoskeletal: reactive arthritis

PATHOGENESIS

Induces inflammation

EPIDEMIOLOGY

Transmission:
  Trachoma: direct contact, fomites, vectors (such as flies)
  Inclusion conjunctivitis: genital (primary infection) to hand to eye
  Genital chlamydia and LGV: sexual contact
  Neonatal: vertical—usually perinatal
Trachoma is the leading cause of infectious blindness worldwide; high incidence in Africa

DIAGNOSIS

Culture: does not grow in artificial media—use live cell culture
  In cell culture—large, cytoplasmic inclusions within epithelial cells will be seen (3) and iodine may be used to better visualize inclusions
Nucleic acid amplification tests (NAATs)—dual testing for *C. trachomatis* and *Neisseria gonorrhoeae* is recommended.

TREATMENT

Depends on infection type

Doxycycline and azithromycin are generally effective

Note: Because 50% of patients are co-infected with gonorrhea and chlamydia, the CDC recommends dual treatment for both pathogens; hence azithromycin plus ceftriaxone may be used

Explanation 1: *Chlamydia trachomatis* serovars D–K are sexually transmitted and cause infections in both adults and neonates. Neonatal infections of the eye, also called ophthalmia neonatorum, are usually a result of transmission from an infected mother during birth and occur 5 to 14 days after birth. This is in contrast to *Neisseria gonorrhoeae* neonatal eye infections, which usually occur within in the first 24 to 48 hours following birth. *C. trachomatis* is intracellular, and a key microscopic clue is the presence of intracellular inclusions. *C. trachomatis* neonatal eye infections can be treated with erythromycin or azithromycin.

Explanation 2: *C. trachomatis* serovars D-K are sexually transmitted and cause infections in both adults and neonates. Urogenital infections in males usually manifest as urethritis and in females, cervicitis. In both cases, mucopurulent, clear or in some cases purulent discharge is present. In females, one of the key features of infections with this organism (as well as *Neisseria gonorrhoeae*) is the possibility of pelvic inflammatory disease (PID). *C. trachomatis* is intracellular and needs live cells to grow and is too small to be observed with a Gram stain/light microscopy. The primary treatment for urogenital infections is doxycycline or azithromycin. However, since many individuals are also infected with *N. gonorrhoeae*, it is recommended that ceftriaxone, also be included in the treatment regimen.

Micro gem: While *Gardnerella vaginalis* is frequently implicated in bacterial vaginosis, it is important to note that several pathogens, both anaerobic and aerobic, may play a role in causing bacterial vaginosis.

Vignette: A sexually active 40-year-old woman presents to her primary care physician with vaginal discharge of 1-week duration. She denies vaginal pruritus, irritation, and pelvic or abdominal pain. Physical exam is normal except for the discharge, which appears thin and creamish and has a foul smell. A vaginal swab is collected and sent to the laboratory for further testing. The whiff test performed on the vaginal discharge is positive, and the vaginal pH is 4.9. No WBCs are present in the wet preparation from the discharge.

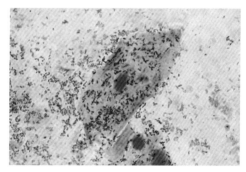

(1)

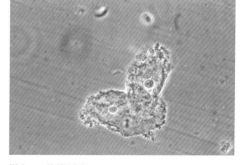

(2) *Source:* CDC/M. Rein
CDC public health library PHIL (phil.cdc.gov) image No. 3720
(http://phil.cdc.gov/phil/details_linked.asp?pid=3720)

DESCRIPTION

Gram-positive rod (may be gram-variable and stain both pink and purple), pleomorphic

"Clue cells" (1,2) may be present—large, desquamated epithelial cells with bacteria attached to edges and inside of cells

INFECTIONS

PRIMARY

Reproductive: bacterial vaginosis (BV)—asymptomatic or thin, off-white discharge with "fishy smell"

PATHOGENESIS

Vagolysin: pore-forming toxin

EPIDEMIOLOGY

Transmission: infections arise following alterations of vaginal microbiota, which facilitates overgrowth of *G. vaginalis* (endogenous strains)

Risk factors: new/increased sexual partners, douching

DIAGNOSIS

Clue cells: squamous epithelial cells with gram-positive rods attached

Amsel criteria (two out of three must be present):
1. thin off-white discharge;
2. vaginal pH > 4.5;
3. positive whiff test (10% KOH plus vaginal fluid = fishy odor)

TREATMENT

Oral: metronidazole

Intravaginal: metronidazole, clindamycin

Explanation: This is a case of bacterial vaginosis (BV). Although BV is classically associated with the facultative anaerobe *Gardnerella vaginalis,* other bacterial pathogens including the anaerobe *Mobiluncus* are also agents of BV. BV occurs after a loss of the normal vaginal microbiota, especially lactobacilli. When lactobacilli levels decrease, the vaginal pH increases (normal vaginal pH = 3.5 to 4.6) which results in an overgrowth of other bacteria, including *Gardnerella* and anaerobes. Anaerobes produce enzymes that break down vaginal peptides into amines. Amines are malodorous; hence, the discharge in BV is often malodorous and described as "fishy."

Micro gem: The agents of genital ulcer disease include *Haemophilus ducreyi,* ●100, *Chlamydia trachomatis* ●, serotypes L1, L2, and L3 (lymphogranuloma venereum), ●103, *Klebsiella granulomatis* (granuloma inguinale) ●, ●106, *Treponema pallidum* ●, and ●139, Herpes simplex virus (HSV)-1 and -2 ●.

Vignette: A 44-year-old man presents with a painful sore on his penis. He recently returned from a trip to South Sudan and indicates that he participated in unprotected sexual activity while abroad. His temperature is 37.1°C (98.8°F). Physical examination reveals four ulcers on the glans penis and prepuce. The base of the ulcers contains purulent material. Inguinal lymphadenopathy is pronounced, and buboes are present.

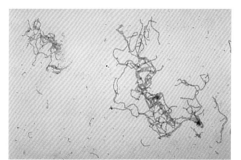

(1) *Source:* CDC/Dr. Greg Hammond
CDC public health library PHIL (phil.cdc.gov) image No. 2775
(http://phil.cdc.gov/phil/details_linked.asp?pid=2775)

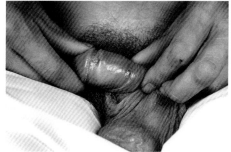

(2) *Source:* CDC/Dr. Pirozzi
CDC public health library PHIL (phil.cdc.gov) image No. 15567
(http://phil.cdc.gov/phil/details_linked.asp?pid=15567)

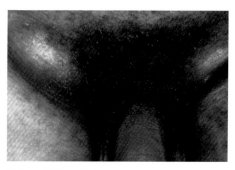

(3) *Source:* CDC/Susan Lindsey
CDC public health library PHIL (phil.cdc.gov) image No. 5821
(http://phil.cdc.gov/phil/details_linked.asp?pid=5821)

DESCRIPTION　Gram-negative coccobacilli (1); may be arranged in "school of fish" formation

INFECTIONS
PRIMARY　Reproductive: chancroid (2)—starts as papule, most often on genitals; progresses to painful, soft ulcer; inguinal lymphadenopathy that may enlarge to form buboes (3)

EPIDEMIOLOGY　Transmission: sexual contact
Geographic distribution: not common in U.S.; higher incidence in areas of Africa, Caribbean, and Southeast Asia

DIAGNOSIS　Culture—good growth on chocolate agar; needs X factor (hemin) to grow; chocolate agar is supplemented with X and V factors (nicotinamide adenine dinucleotide (NAD))
See also ● 130, *Haemophilus influenzae* ●

TREATMENT　Azithromycin, ceftriaxone

Explanation: This man most likely has chancroid caused by the gram-negative coccobacillus *Haemophilus ducreyi*. Chancroid starts as an erythematous papule that develops into a pustule and then a soft, painful ulcer/chancre with ragged edges. Often multiple lesions are present and inguinal lymphadenopathy and buboes may be seen. Chancroid is more common in sub-Saharan Africa and Southeast Asia than in the United States.

Vignette: A 57-year-old Nigerian man visits his village clinic with a sore on his penis. He claims it does not hurt, but his partner wanted him to have a doctor look at it prior to engaging in sexual activity. Vital signs are normal, and physical examination shows the presence of two bright red ulcers on the penis. Inguinal lymphadenopathy is not present.

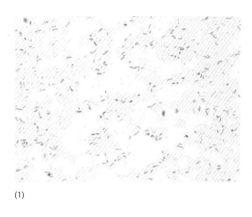

(1)

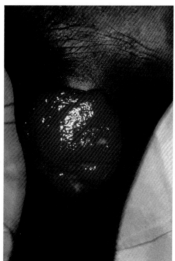

(2) *Source:* CDC/Joe Miller; slides provided by Dr. Tabua, chief
medical officer from Port Moresby, Papua, New Guinea
CDC public health library PHIL (phil.cdc.gov) image No. 5364
(http://phil.cdc.gov/phil/details_linked.asp?pid=5364)

DESCRIPTION

Gram-negative rod (1); part of *Enterobacteriaceae* family
See also ● 129, *Escherichia coli* ●; ● 131, *Klebsiella pneumoniae* ●; ● 97, *Proteus* ●; ● 47, *Salmonella enterica* serotype typhi and paratyphi ●; ● 70, Nontyphoidal *Salmonella* ●; ● 71, *Shigella* ●; ● 74, *Yersinia enterocolitica* and *pseudotuberculosis* ●; ● 138, *Yersinia pestis* ●

INFECTIONS

PRIMARY

Reproductive: granuloma inguinale (Donovanosis)—"beefy red," firm, painless ulcers (2); inguinal lymphadenopathy not usually present; pseudobuboes present

PATHOGENESIS

Capsule
Intracellular—lives within macrophages
See also ● 121, *Leishmania* ●; ● 37, *Histoplasma capsulatum* ●

EPIDEMIOLOGY

Transmission: sexual contact
Geographic distribution: rare in the U.S.; more common in tropical countries

DIAGNOSIS

Microscopy: scrapings or biopsy from culture will show Donovan bodies which are rod shaped bacteria within the cytoplasm of monocytes, macrophages, and histocytes

TREATMENT

Doxycycline

Explanation: This man has an infection with *Klebsiella granulomatis*, a gram-negative rod. In this infection, firm, painless nodules or papules form at the site of inoculation. These eventually ulcerate. The ulcers are highly vascular and bleed easily, giving a "beefy" red appearance. Although lymphadenopathy is not usually present, pseudobuboes (subcutaneous granulomas) may be present. Identification of Donovan bodies from the ulcer aids in diagnosis. Donovan bodies are rod-shaped bacteria within the cytoplasm of monocytes, macrophages, and histocytes.
See also ● 139, Herpes simplex virus (HSV)-1 and -2 ●; ● 102, *Haemophilus ducreyi* ●; ● 100, *Chlamydia trachomatis* ●; ● 106, *Treponema pallidum* ●

Vignette: A 53-year-old man presents with a 3-day history of painful urination. He denies penile or urethral discharge. He is sexually active with one female partner. His vital signs are unremarkable. On examination, the urethral meatus is inflamed, and clear discharge is present after gentle stripping of the penis. Gram stain from the discharge is reported as many PMNs and no organisms are seen. Nucleic acid amplification tests (NAATs) for *N. gonorrhoeae* and *C. trachomatis* are negative.

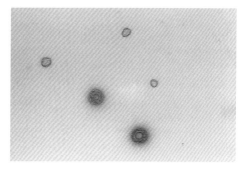

(1) *Source:* CDC/Dr. E. Arum; Dr. N. Jacobs
    CDC public health library PHIL (phil.cdc.gov) image No. 1021
    (http://phil.cdc.gov/phil/details_linked.asp?pid=11021)

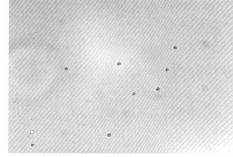

(2) *Source:* CDC/Dr. Frances Forrester
    CDC public health library PHIL (phil.cdc.gov) image No. 10930
    (http://phil.cdc.gov/phil/details_linked.asp?pid=10930)

DESCRIPTION

No cell wall
Does not Gram stain
Very tiny
Mycoplasma: cell membrane contains sterols (cholesterol)
Clinically important species: *M. hominis, M genitalium* (1), *U. urealyticum* (2)

INFECTIONS

PRIMARY

Renal/urinary: UTIs
Reproductive: nongonococcal urethritis, cervicitis (which may possibly result in pelvic inflammatory disease [PID])

OTHER

Skin and soft tissue: wounds
Systemic: postpartum bacteremia
Neonatal:
    Nervous: meningitis
    Respiratory: pneumonia
    Systemic: bacteremia

PATHOGENESIS

Ureaplasma: urease—breaks down urea and produces ammonia
PUNCH = Urease positive organisms
● 97, *Proteus mirabilis* ●; ● *Ureaplasma* ●; ● 28, *Nocardia* ●;
● 11, *Cryptococcus neoformans* and *gatti* ●; ● 69, *Heliobacter pylori* ●

EPIDEMIOLOGY

May colonize urogenital tract of healthy adults
Transmission:
    Post-natal: displacement of endogenous strains
    Neonatal: vertical—most often perinatal

DIAGNOSIS

Culture: *Mycoplasma* requires serum for growth
PCR

TREATMENT

Adults: doxycycline, azithromycin

Explanation: Urethritis in males may be asymptomatic, but the most common manifestation is dysuria, as presented in this case. Several pathogens are involved in urethritis in males, most notably ● 105, *Neisseria gonorrhoeae* ●, *C. trachomatis*, *U. urealyticum*, and *M. hominis*. *N. gonorrhoeae* may be seen on a Gram stain as intracellular and extracellular gram-negative diplococci. Because the Gram stain did not show organisms resembling *N. gonorrhoeae*, this is probably a case of non-gonococcal urethritis. Because the nucleic acid amplification test (NAAT) is negative for *C. trachomatis*, the etiologic agent of this infection is likely *Ureaplasma* or *Mycoplasma*.

Vignette: A 35-year-old man presents with penile discharge and dysuria. The previous week he had attended an all-weekend party with some friends and does not recall the details of what occurred, but he does remember meeting many women and may have participated in unprotected sex. On examination, he is afebrile, and a purulent penile discharge is observed. A Gram stain from the discharge demonstrates many white blood cells and many intracellular and extracellular gram-negative diplococci.

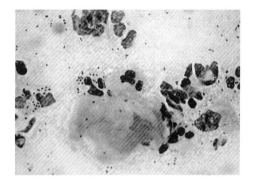

(1)

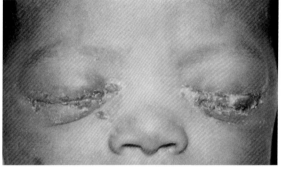

(2) *Source:* CDC/J. Pledger
CDC public health library PHIL (phil.cdc.gov) image No. 3766
(http://phil.cdc.gov/phil/details_linked.asp?pid=3766)

DESCRIPTION

Gram-negative diplococci, kidney/coffee bean–shaped (1)
Characteristic gram-negative diplococci (GNDC) with PMNs (both intracellular and extracellular).
See also ●4, *Neisseria meningitidis* ●; ●16, *Moraxella catarrhalis* ●
Alternative name: gonococcus (GC)

INFECTIONS

PRIMARY

Reproductive: genital gonorrhea—asymptomatic or symptomatic cervicitis
Complications: pelvic inflammatory disease (PID)—associated with Fitz-Hugh–Curtis syndrome; prostatitis, epididymitis, urethritis
Neonatal:
Head and neck: eye—conjunctivitis (ophthalmia neonatorum) (2)—24 to 48 hours after birth

OTHER

Head and neck
Eye—hyperacute bacterial conjunctivitis in adults
Pharynx—pharyngitis
Post-infectious sequelae: septic arthritis

PATHOGENESIS

Endotoxin/lipooligosaccharide (LOS)—similar function as LPS
Pili: capable of phase and antigenic variation
Outer membrane proteins: opacity (opa) proteins—assist in adhesion—capable of phase and antigenic variation
IgA protease—destroys IgA
See also ●130, *Haemophilus influenzae* ●; ●4, *Neisseria meningitidis* ●; ●136, *Streptococcus pneumoniae* ●

EPIDEMIOLOGY

Transmission:
Genital gonorrhea, pharyngitis: sexual contact
Neonatal: vertical—usually perinatal
Hyperacute bacterial conjunctivitis: genital (primary infection) to hand to eye

DIAGNOSIS

Culture: best growth on chocolate agar or selective media such as Thayer-Martin; carbohydrate utilization test—glucose oxidizer.
See also ●4, *Neisseria meningitidis* ●
Gram stain: intracellular and extracellular GNDC on a Gram stain from a male urogenital specimen is indicative of GC; however, this is not the case for female urogenital specimens because females may have normal non-gonococcal *Neisseria* species in the urogenital tract
Nucleic acid amplification tests (NAATs)—dual testing for ●100, *Chlamydia trachomatis* ● and *Neisseria gonorrhoeae* is recommended.

TREATMENT

Ceftriaxone (recommended for both urogenital and neonatal eye infections)
Notes: This pathogen exhibits increasing antimicrobial resistance. Because 50% of patients are co-infected with gonorrhea and chlamydia, the CDC recommends dual treatment for both pathogens; hence azithromycin plus ceftriaxone may be used

ANIMATIONS

http://go.thieme.com/microb/Video105.1

Explanation: *Neisseria gonorrhoeae*, a gram-negative diplococcus, is also called gonococcus. It is involved in sexually transmitted infections (STIs), disseminated infections, notably arthritis, and newborn conjunctivitis. In males, the typical Gram stain shows gram-negative diplococci within neutrophils. Because females have normal *Neisseria* species that may be part of the vaginal microbiota, a Gram stain finding of gram-negative diplococci is not necessarily indicative of genital gonorrhea.

Micro gem: The rash of secondary syphilis may be seen on the palms and soles. Other infections with rashes on the palms and soles include rickettsia (● 46, *Rickettsia* ●) and hand-foot and mouth disease (Coxsackie virus) (● 140, Non-polio enterovirus ●).

Vignette 1: A 23-year-old man visits his physician because of a sore on his penis. He states the sore does not hurt, but he is concerned because it has been present for about 2 weeks. He has not traveled outside of the United States recently. His temperature is 37.1°C (98.8°F), and his pulse is 85 bpm. Physical examination reveals a single, indurated ulcer with demarcated edges on the penile shaft. No urethral discharge is noted. Mild inguinal lymphadenopathy is observed and the lymph nodes are firm and nontender.

Vignette 2: A 46-year-old woman complains of a 1-week history of extreme exhaustion, headache, fever, sore throat, and loss of appetite. She states she was concerned when she noticed a rash on her body, which she claims is not itchy. Her temperature is 38.1°C (100.6°F). Her pharynx is erythematous, and no exudate is seen. Her cervical lymph nodes are enlarged, firm, and nontender. A diffuse maculopapular rash is present on her trunk, back, palms, and soles. The physician decides to do a pelvic exam, and smooth, hypopigmented papules are seen on the skin in the inner thigh and perianal region.

Vignette 3: A woman brings her 67-year-old father to the physician because of increasing forgetfulness and paranoia. She states that he also seems to be more clumsy than usual, especially at night. The man has no prior history of psychosis. Physical examination reveals sensory ataxia. He is oriented to time and place, but has deficits in short-term memory.

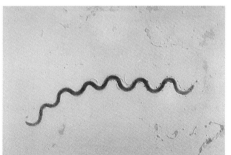

(1) *Source:* CDC/Susan Lindsey
CDC public health library PHIL (phil.cdc.gov)
image No. 14969
(http://phil.cdc.gov/phil/details_linked.
asp?pid=14969)

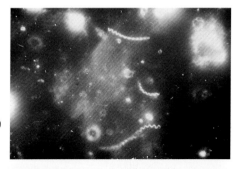

(2) *Source:* CDC/Susan Lindsey
CDC public health library PHIL (phil.cdc.gov)
image No. 1248
(http://phil.cdc.gov/phil/details_linked.
asp?pid=1248)

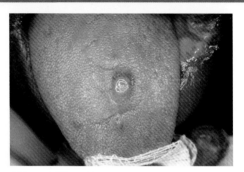

(3) *Source:* CDC/Robert E. Sumpter
   CDC public health library PHIL (phil.cdc.gov) image No. 12623
   (http://phil.cdc.gov/phil/details_linked.asp?pid=12623)

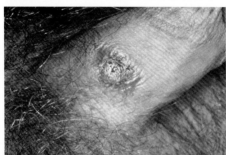

(4) *Source:* CDC/Dr. N. J. Fiumara
   CDC public health library PHIL (phil.cdc.gov)
   image No. 6758
   (http://phil.cdc.gov/phil/details_linked.
   asp?pid=6758)

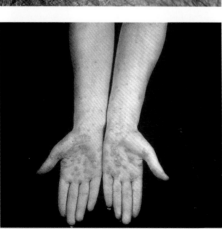

(5) *Source:* CDC/Robert Sumpter
   CDC public health library PHIL (phil.cdc.gov)
   image No. 12587
   (http://phil.cdc.gov/phil/details_linked.
   asp?pid=12587)

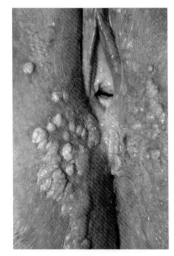

(6) *Source:* CDC/Joyce Ayers
   CDC public health library PHIL (phil.cdc.gov) image
   No. 11256
   (http://phil.cdc.gov/phil/details_linked.asp?pid=11256)

DESCRIPTION

Spirochete (1)
Gram-negative cell wall—outer membrane and LPS
Does not Gram stain well
Dark-field microscopy may be used to visualize (2), but is no longer commonly utilized

INFECTIONS
PRIMARY

Reproductive: syphilis
Primary: painless, hard ulcer/chancre (3,4); inguinal lymphadenopathy may be present
See also ●102, *Haemophilus ducreyi*●; ●103, *Klebsiella granulomatis*●; ●139, Herpes simplex virus (HSV)-1 and -2●; ●100, *Chlamydia trachomatis*●
Secondary (disseminated): maculopapular rash (on palms and soles) (5), generalized lymphadenopathy, meningitis, condylomata lata (6)
Tertiary: neurosyphilis (tabes dorsalis, general paresis), cardiovascular (involves aorta), gummas
Congenital: stillbirth, neonatal death, facial abnormalities (saddle nose), Hutchinson teeth, hearing loss

TORCH = congenital infections
●**T**oxoplasma gondii●; **O**ther (*Treponema pallidum*, ●117, Varicella-zoster virus●, ●55, Parvovirus B19●); ●142, **R**ubella virus●; ●48, **C**ytomegalovirus (CMV)●; ●139, **H**erpes simplex virus (HSV)-1 and -2●

EPIDEMIOLOGY

Transmission:
Post-natal infections:
Sexual contact
Direct contact with chancre
Blood transfusion (rare)
Congenital: vertical—usually *in utero*

DIAGNOSIS

Dark-field microscopy from chancre or condylomata lata demonstrating spirochetes
Serology
Non-treponema/screening tests: detect regain antibodies to cardiolipin antigen
Note: False positive may be caused by HIV, HSV, RA, SLE, pregnancy and other conditions, hence these test are not specific and are screening assays
• RPR (rapid plasma reagin)
• VDRL (Venereal Disease Research Laboratory)
• TRUST (toluidine red unheated serum test)
Treponema tests/confirmatory tests: detect antibodies to *T. pallidum*
• FTA-ABS (fluorescent *Treponema* antibody-absorption)
• TPHA (*Treponema pallidum* hemagglutination)
• TP-PA (*Treponema* particle agglutination)
• MHA-TP (microhemagglutination *Treponema pallidum*)
In the past, non-treponema tests screening non-treponema tests were first performed. If positive results were confirmed by *Treponema* specific (antibody) tests. If negative, repeat testing in 3-months was recommended.
The CDC currently recommends testing first with EIA or chemiluminescence assays (CIA). This should then be followed with the RPR, and if positive, syphilis can be confirmed. However, if the RPR is negative, then *Treponema* specific (antibody) tests must be performed. If positive, a diagnosis of syphilis can be confirmed. If negative, syphilis is unlikely.

TREATMENT

Penicillin G
Jarisch-Herxheimer reaction may occur

Explanation 1: This is a case of primary syphilis, a sexually transmitted infection caused by *Treponema pallidum*, a spirochete-shaped bacteria. Spirochetes are best visualized with dark-field microscopy. The chancre or ulcer of primary syphilis may go unnoticed because it is painless and is self-resolving. The chancre is usually indurated (hard) with well-defined edges. With primary syphilis, genital exudate is usually absent, but mild to moderate inguinal lymphadenopathy may be present.

Explanation 2: This patient has secondary syphilis caused by the spirochete *Treponema pallidum*. The stages of syphilis are denoted as primary, secondary, and tertiary. Syphilis may be latent as well. Typical findings of secondary syphilis include a nonpruritic, bilaterally symmetrical, maculopapular rash on the trunk, back, and extremities, including the palms and soles, generalized lymphadenopathy, "flu-like" symptoms, alopecia, and condylomata lata. Condylomata lata are smooth, flat papules that are generally painless. They are usually found on the genitals, perianal region, and other areas that are moist. Other findings of secondary syphilis include central nervous system (CNS) abnormalities and ocular abnormalities.

Explanation 3: The patient has symptoms of neurosyphilis. Neurosyphilis occurs 5 to 30 years after the initial exposure and may affect any organ system including the nervous system, cardiovascular system, and skin. Manifestations of neurosyphilis may include meningitis, dementia, psychosis, general paresis, and tabes dorsalis. Because primary syphilis presents as a painless genital ulcer, patients may or may not remember the initial genital infection. The FTA-ABS is usually positive, which would aid in confirming the diagnosis. FTA-ABS is a treponema-specific test that can be used in the diagnosis of late syphilis. Non-treponema tests, such as RPR, may be negative in late syphilis.

Vignette: A 54-year-old man who has sex with men presents with a mass on his perianal region. He states the mass is itchy, tender, and burns, but does not hurt. His vital signs are unremarkable. Physical examination of the anus reveals pink verrucous lesions. The VDRL is nonreactive.

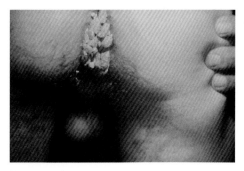

(1) *Source:* CDC/Dr. Weisner
    CDC public health library PHIL (phil.cdc.gov) image No. 4151
    (http://phil.cdc.gov/phil/details_linked.asp?pid=4151)

DESCRIPTION

Taxonomy: Papillomavirus family
Virus properties: double-stranded DNA, non-enveloped
> 100 types of HPV

INFECTIONS

PRIMARY

Types 6 and 11 (and others)
  Reproductive: condyloma acuminatum (anogenital warts) (1)
Types 1, 2, 3, 4, 7, and 10 (and others)
  Skin and soft tissue: warts—common, plantar, flat, and butcher's wart

OTHER

Neonatal: recurrent respiratory papillomatosis (laryngeal tumors)

PATHOGENESIS

Increased risk of cervical and penile cancer, head/neck/oral tumors; some strains inactivate the tumor suppressor genes *p53* and *Rb*

EPIDEMIOLOGY

Transmission:
  Condyloma acuminatum: sexual contact
  Warts: close contact or contact with contaminated skin
  Neonatal: vertical—usually perinatal
High risk: highest risk of cervical cancer when infected with types 16 and 18

DIAGNOSIS

Cytology/pap smear: for cervical cancer screening; HPV infected squamous epithelial cells appear koilocytotic
PCR
Genotyping

PREVENTION

Vaccine: recombinant vaccines—Gardasil (types 6, 11, 16, and 18), Gardasil 9 (same as Gardasil plus types 31, 33, 45, 52, and 58), Cervarix (types 16 and 18)

TREATMENT

Supportive; keratolytic agents and immune-mediated therapies

Explanation: The is a case of genital warts or condyloma acuminata, which is caused by human papillomavirus (HPV), a double-stranded DNA virus. These skin-colored or pink warts are often described as verrucous or cauliflower like. Condyloma acuminata is a sexually transmitted infection and men who have sex with men are more prone to warts in the perianal area. Certain strains of HPV, including types 16 and 18, increase the risk of neoplasia.

108 Trichomonas vaginalis

Micro gem: The typical agents of vaginitis are *Trichomonas vaginalis* and ● 143, *Candida* species ●.
In contrast, vaginosis is usually bacterial and may involve several pathogens, including ● 101, *Gardnerella vaginalis* ●.

Vignette: A 34-year-old woman presents with vaginal discharge and itchiness of 4 days' duration. She is sexually active and recently started a new relationship. A pelvic exam reveals purulent, green-frothy discharge and vaginal and cervical edema and erythema. A wet preparation from the discharge demonstrates the presence of a motile, pear-shaped organism and many white blood cells.

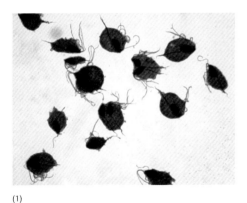

(1)

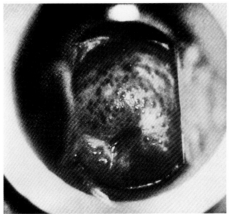

(2) *Source:* CDC public health library PHIL (phil.cdc.gov) image
No. 5240
(http://phil.cdc.gov/phil/details_linked.asp?pid=5240)

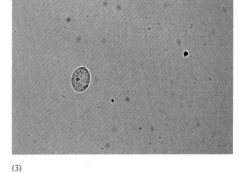

(3)

DESCRIPTION

Protozoa: flagellate
Clinically significant morphological form: trophozoite (1)

INFECTIONS
  PRIMARY

Reproductive:
  Females: vaginitis—pruritus, cervical erythema [strawberry cervix (2)], thin, green, malodorous discharge; increased vaginal pH
  Males: mostly asymptomatic, urethritis

EPIDEMIOLOGY

Transmission: sexual

DIAGNOSIS

Wet preparation: identification of pear-shaped trophozoite (3); jerky motility; WBCs present
  The sensitivity of the wet prep is quite low, hence negative results should be followed up with additional testing
Nucleic acid amplification tests (NAATs): more sensitive for the detection of *T. vaginalis* than the wet prep

TREATMENT

Metronidazole, tinidazole

ANIMATION

http://go.thieme.com/microb/Video108.1

Explanation: *Trichomonas vaginalis* is a pear-shaped protozoan. The organism has characteristic jerky motion and moves via flagella. The motility can be visualized on a wet mount (also referred to as wet preparation). Many females are asymptomatic, but the primary clinical manifestation is vaginitis. Findings include purulent thin, green-frothy discharge, vulvar irritation, pruritus, dysuria, and dyspareunia. Erythema is often pronounced, and the cervix is described as "strawberry cervix" (punctate hemorrhage) due to mucosal capillary dilation. White blood cells are most often present as well. Symptoms of infection are often worse during menses.

Micro gem: A hallmark of cutaneous anthrax is an eschar. Other infections in which an eschar may also be present include tularemia (● 111, *Francisella tularensis* ●), cutaneous diphtheria (● 17, *Corynebacterium diphtheriae* ●), and scrub typhus (*Orientia tsutsugamushi*) (● 46, *Rickettsia* ●).

Vignette: A 62-year-old man presents to his primary care physician with a painless black lesion on his right hand. The man states that he works in a factory that processes various animal hides and sheep wool. At the time of the examination, his temperature is 37.2°C (99.0°F), and his physical examination is unremarkable. A sporulated gram-positive rod is observed on a Gram stain from the lesion.

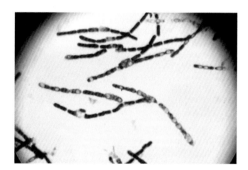

(1) *Source:* CDC public health library PHIL (phil.cdc.gov) image No. 9826
(http://phil.cdc.gov/phil/details_linked.asp?pid=9826)

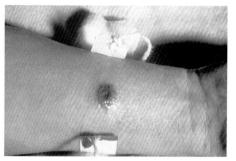

(2) *Source:* CDC public health library PHIL (phil.cdc.gov) image No. 1933
(http://phil.cdc.gov/phil/details_linked.asp?pid=1933)

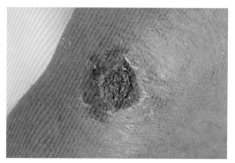

(3) *Source:* CDC/James H. Steel
CDC public health library PHIL (phil.cdc.gov) image No. 2033
(http://phil.cdc.gov/phil/details_linked.asp?pid=2033)

DESCRIPTION

Gram-positive rods (1) with large flattened ends; may form long chains
Spore-producer

INFECTIONS

PRIMARY

Skin and soft tissue (most common): cutaneous anthrax (2,3)
Lesion progression: papule to vesicle/bullae to painless necrotic ulcer with black eschar
Respiratory: inhalation anthrax (also called woolsorter's disease—due to transmission of disease following inhalation of spores in contaminated sheep's wool)

OTHER

Gastrointestinal (rare): diarrhea

PATHOGENESIS

Capsule: unique because it is composed of poly-D-glutamic acid
Exotoxin with three components:
Protective antigen (PA): binds to receptor
Edema factor (EF): increases cAMP, resulting in edema
See also ● 73, *Vibrio cholerae* ●; ● 23, *Bordetella pertussis* ●; ● 68, Enterotoxigenic *Escherichia coli* ●; ● 61, *Bacillus cereus* ●
Lethal factor (LF): protease that decreases MAP kinase, resulting in apoptosis

EPIDEMIOLOGY

Transmission:
Skin and soft tissue: direct contact with spores—zoonotic and commonly associated with herbivores, such as goats and sheep
Respiratory: inhalation of spores
Gastrointestinal: foodborne—ingestion of spores from contaminated meat

DIAGNOSIS

Culture: catalase positive, nonhemolytic, nonmotile—the latter two test differentiate this organism from other *Bacillus* species
Appropriate safety precautions must be followed when working with this organism
Immunohistochemical staining
PCR

PREVENTION

Vaccination of animals and high-risk individuals, such as military, laboratory personnel
Anthrax vaccine absorbed (Biothrax): contains cell free filtrate from attenuated, avirulent *B. anthracis*—blocks PA

TREATMENT

Depends on type of infection
Inhalation anthrax: antibiotic plus antitoxin OR antibiotic plus immunoglobulin
Antibiotic: ciprofloxacin, doxycycline, clindamycin
Antitoxin: raxibacumab, obiltoxaximab—inhibit PA

Explanation: *Bacillus anthracis* is an aerobic gram-positive rod with spores. This pathogen is often associated with contact with hides or wool from sheep and goats. Infections may also be transmitted from inhalation of spores. *B. anthracis* causes three main type of infections: (1) pulmonary anthrax, also called Woolsorter's disease; (2) cutaneous anthrax, which starts as a red, itchy bump, but progresses to a painless black ulcer; and (3) gastrointestinal anthrax, which is quite rare.

Micro gem: *Clostridium perfringens* is an agent of necrotizing fasciitis. Other agents of necrotizing fasciitis include anaerobic pathogens such as ● 124, *Bacteroides* ● and aerobic pathogens, especially ● 135, *Streptococcus pyogenes* ● and *Enterobacteriaceae*, including ● 129, *Escherichia coli* ●, ● 131, *Klebsiella pneumoniae* ●, and ● 97, *Proteus mirabilis* ●.

Vignette 1: A 23-year-old medical student wakes up in the middle of the night with abdominal pain, cramping, and watery diarrhea. He has four bowel movements within 3 hours. He doesn't notice any blood in his stool and he doesn't feel feverish and is not vomiting. While on clerkships the previous day, he ate in the hospital cafeteria, which was celebrating Thanksgiving. He recalls eating turkey, stuffing, mashed potatoes, and gravy and green beans. By early afternoon of the next day he is feeling better. Later it is discovered that several other hospital employees were also ill following the same meal. A toxin from an anaerobic gram-positive rod is identified from the tainted food.

Vignette 2: A 25-year-old man is hospitalized following a motor vehicle accident. Approximately 24 hours following admission, he experiences severe pain in his leg. The skin of the affected leg appears purple. Later that evening, overlying bullae are apparent on the leg. Physical exam reveals crepitus, and radiographic imaging demonstrates the presence of gas within the soft tissue.

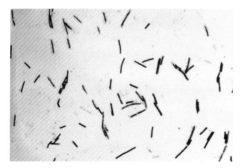

(1) *Source:* CDC/Don Stalons
CDC public health library PHIL (phil.cdc.gov) image No. 2995
(http://phil.cdc.gov/phil/details_linked.asp?pid=2995)

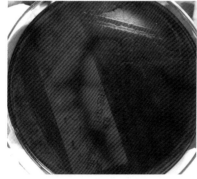

(2)

(3) *Source:* CDC/Dr. Stuart E. Starr
CDC public health library PHIL (phil.cdc.gov) image No. 3873
(http://phil.cdc.gov/phil/details_linked.asp?pid=3873)

DESCRIPTION
Gram-positive rods (1), large, box-car shaped
Spore-producer
Obligate anaerobe
Types A to E; type A is the most clinically significant pathogen

INFECTIONS
PRIMARY
Gastrointestinal: enteritis—watery diarrhea and necrotizing enteritis (pigbel)
Skin and soft tissue/musculoskeletal: cellulitis, necrotizing fasciitis, myonecrosis (gas gangrene)

OTHER
Systemic: bacteremia
Reproductive: endometritis

PATHOGENESIS
Exotoxins: *C. perfringens* types A to E—each produces a different toxin
  Type A—alpha toxin (also called lecithinase)—phospholipase that hydrolyzes lecithin and sphingomyelin; results in disruption of membrane of RBCs, WBCs and other cells
    Contributes to skin and soft tissue infections
Enterotoxin: disrupts selective permeability of the plasma membrane and leads to cell death
  Contributes to GI infections

EPIDEMIOLOGY
Found in soil and water
Transmission:
  Foodborne: ingestion of spores that produce toxin *in vivo*
    Enteritis—commonly associated foods include beef, poultry, gravy, dried precooked foods
    Pigbel—pork (pig intestines)
  Skin and soft tissue: contact with bacteria or spores following trauma to skin/tissue

High risk for skin and soft tissue infections: trauma to the skin, such as wounds that develop following gunshot, bowel surgery, intramuscular injection

DIAGNOSIS
Culture: anaerobic growth with double zone of beta-hemolysis (2), lecithinase positive on egg yolk agar (3)
Toxin detection

TREATMENT
For non-foodborne infections: penicillin G plus clindamycin

Explanation 1: The etiological agent of this infection is the anaerobic gram-positive rod, *Clostridium perfringens*. This pathogen is a spore-producer and the spores are heat-resistant. When food is rewarmed or when food is not refrigerated, the vegetative form of the spores can multiply. Commonly associated foods include gravies, stews, soups, beef, poultry and pre-cooked foods. *In vivo* an enterotoxin, which forms pores in enterocytes, is produced. The toxin increases membrane permeability, which leads to diarrhea and loss of fluids. The incubation is approximately 8–24 hours after the ingestion of contaminated food. Typical symptoms include nausea, abdominal pain and watery diarrhea. Infections with this pathogen may be hard to differentiate from diarrheal infections with ●61, *Bacillus cereus* ●, which is an aerobic gram-positive rod.

Explanation 2: Gas gangrene or myonecrosis is an acute infection that results in destruction of muscle tissue. One of the main causative agents is *Clostridium perfringens*. The pathogen produces exotoxins that contribute to tissue injury. *C. perfringens*, an obligate anaerobe, is a gram-positive rod.

Vignette: A 12-year-old boy presents with fever, chills, and headache of 3 days' duration. The previous weekend he went hiking with the Boy Scouts and had moved a dead rabbit from the trail. The boy's temperature is 38.8°C (101.8°F). On examination, a small ulcer with a raised border and black base is seen on his right index finger. The epitrochlear lymph nodes on his right arm are swollen. Serological tests confirm the presence of *Francisella tularensis*. Regional lymph nodes are often enlarged.

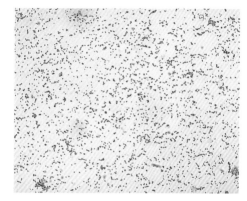

(1) *Source:* CDC/Courtesy of Larry Stauffer, Oregon State Public Health Laboratory
CDC public health library PHIL (phil.cdc.gov) image No. 1901
(http://phil.cdc.gov/phil/details_linked.asp?pid=1901)

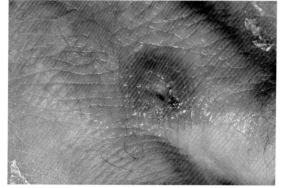

(2) *Source:* CDC/Dr. Brachman
CDC public health library PHIL (phil.cdc.gov) image No. 2037
(http://phil.cdc.gov/phil/details_linked.asp?pid=2037)

DESCRIPTION	Gram-negative coccobacilli (1)
INFECTION PRIMARY	Tularemia Skin and soft tissue (most common): ulceroglandular (2)—cutaneous ulcer with lymphadenopathy; eschar may form at site of inoculation Lymphatic: glandular—regional lymphadenopathy
OTHER	Head and Neck: eye—oculoglandular—red, swollen eyes with possible ulcer Respiratory: oropharyngeal infections, pneumonia Systemic: typhoidal, septic forms of infection
PATHOGENESIS	Capsule Facultative intracellular pathogen

EPIDEMIOLOGY	Zoonotic: reservoirs include wild rodents, rabbits, beavers, domestic cats
	Transmission:
	  Contact with contaminated animal
	  Bite of arthropod—usually tick
	  Ingestion of contaminated food and water
	  Inhalation

DIAGNOSIS	Culture: slow grower; needs cysteine to grow Appropriate safety precautions must be followed when working with this organism Serology: antibody detection (most common method of diagnosis) PCR—not widely available
TREATMENT	Moderate or serious infections: streptomycin Milder infections: ciprofloxacin, doxycycline

Explanation: This boy has ulceroglandular tularensis caused by *Francisella tularensis*. The ulcer on his finger is an eschar which most often forms at the site of inoculation. *F. tularensis* is a zoonotic intracellular gram-negative coccobacillus. Commonly associated animals include small rodents and rabbits. This pathogen can also be transmitted by the bite of a tick, ingestion and inhalation. Depending on the mechanism of transmission, different clinical manifestations may be observed. The most common form is ulceroglandular tularemia as described in this case, which occurs following a tick bite or contact with an infected animal.

Vignette: A 53-year-old man in rural India visits the local clinic with weakness of his wrist and forearm and several lesions on his skin. On exam, two macular lesions are noted on his left forearm. The man has a decreased sensation in the area of the lesions, and on palpation the ulnar nerve is enlarged.

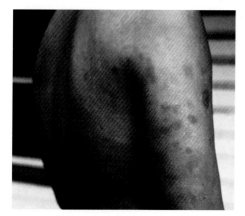

(1) *Source:* CDC/Arthur E. Kaye
CDC public health library PHIL (phil.cdc.gov) image No. 15497
(http://phil.cdc.gov/phil/details_linked.asp?pid=15497)

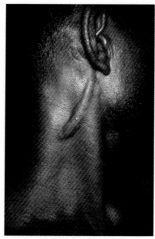

(2) *Source:* CDC/Arthur E. Kaye
CDC public health library PHIL (phil.cdc.gov) image No. 16519
(http://phil.cdc.gov/phil/details_linked.asp?pid=16519)

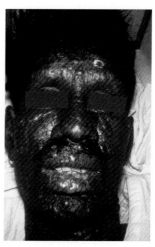

(3) *Source:* CDC/Dr. Andre J. Lebrun
CDC public health library PHIL (phil.cdc.gov) image No. 15508
(http://phil.cdc.gov/phil/details_linked.asp?pid=15508)

DESCRIPTION
Acid-fast bacilli (AFB)
Mycolic acid (a type of fatty acid) in cell wall
Does not Gram stain

INFECTIONS
PRIMARY
Leprosy (also called Hansen's disease)
Skin and soft tissue, nervous system, mucous membranes: macular, papular lesions (1); skin may be hypopigmented; numbness/loss of sensation when lesions are touched
Two main forms of leprosy
Paucibacillary (tuberculoid): milder form; < 5 lesions; peripheral nerve enlargement (2)
Multibacillary (lepromatous): more serious form; > 5 lesions; leonine facies (3) (lion-like face); nerve endings affected; cartilage damage may occur

PATHOGENESIS
Mediated by cell-mediated immunity
Paucibacillary: infected individual able to mount a strong Th1 response to *M. leprae*
Multibacillary: infected individual mounts a minimal Th1 response to *M. leprae* (Th2 response is normal)

EPIDEMIOLOGY
Transmission: most likely via respiratory droplets
Animal reservoir: armadillo
Geographic distribution: increased incidence in tropical areas, especially Asia and Africa

DIAGNOSIS
Usually made on clinical manifestations
Organism cannot be grown *in vitro*
Microscopy: skin biopsy may show AFB
PCR

TREATMENT
Depends on type of leprosy
Paucibacillary: dapsone plus rifampin
Multibacillary: rifampin plus clofazimine

Explanation: Leprosy is not a common infection in the United States. Classic manifestations of leprosy include lesions with a loss of sensation and peripheral nerve involvement. The two main types of leprosy are tuberculoid or paucibacillary leprosy and lepromatous or bacillary leprosy.

Vignette: A 47-year-old woman presents with a 2-day history of a swollen, painful hand following a cat bite. Her temperature is 38.2°C (100.8°F). Two small puncture marks are seen on the dorsal surface of her right hand near the base of the thumb, and small amount of purulent drainage is present. Her right hand is significantly swollen, erythematous, and tender. Red streaks are extending from her infected hand to her elbow. Gram stain from the purulent drainage demonstrates the presence of gram-negative coccobacilli.

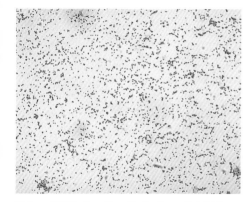

(1) *Source:* CDC/Courtesy of Larry Stauffer, Oregon State Public
Health Laboratory
CDC public health library PHIL (phil.cdc.gov) image No. 1901
(http://phil.cdc.gov/phil/details_linked.asp?pid=1901)

DESCRIPTION   Gram-negative coccobacilli (1) or short rod

INFECTIONS

PRIMARY   Skin and soft tissue: cellulitis, abscesses
Musculoskeletal: septic arthritis, osteomyelitis

OTHER   Respiratory: pharyngitis, pneumonia
Systemic: bacteremia
Cardiovascular: endocarditis

PATHOGENESIS   Capsule
LPS

EPIDEMIOLOGY   Zoonotic: normal oral microbiota of cats and dogs
Transmission: bite or scratch from infected animal (more often cat)
Respiratory infections associated with individuals with underlying pulmonary disease

DIAGNOSIS   Culture: oxidase positive; indole positive; does not grow on MacConkey agar

TREATMENT   Penicillin, amoxicillin

Explanation: *Pasteurella multocida* is part of the normal oral microbiota of cats and dogs and can be transmitted to humans following a bite or scratch from an infected animal. Infections commonly manifest as cellulitis as described in this case, but the infection may progress to the joints, bone, and bloodstream as well. *P. multocida* is a gram-negative coccobacillus.

Micro gem: Classic symptoms of measles are 3C's and a P: **c**ough, **c**oryza, **c**onjunctivitis, and **p**hotophobia

Vignette: An 8-year-old boy presents with a flat, red rash. The child's mother states that 3 days ago the child had a fever, cough, and runny nose. The previous day the mother noticed whitish "spots" on the boy's mouth. She brought him to the emergency department when she noticed the rash. On examination, the boy's temperature is 37.5°C (99.5°F). A blanching, maculopapular rash is noted on his face, neck, trunk, and extremities, but not on the soles and palms. Whitish lesions are noted on the buccal mucosa. The child is not up to date on his immunizations.

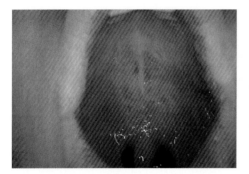

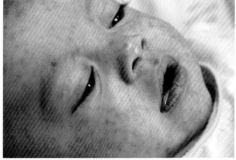

(1) *Source:* CDC/Heinz F. Eichenwald, MD
    CDC public health library PHIL (phil.cdc.gov) image No. 3187
    (http://phil.cdc.gov/phil/details_linked.asp?pid=3187)

(2) *Source:* CDC/Molly Kurnit, MPH
    CDC public health library PHIL (phil.cdc.gov) image No. 19434
    (http://phil.cdc.gov/phil/details_linked.asp?pid=19434)

DESCRIPTION
Taxonomy: Paramyxovirus family; *Morbillivirus* genus
Virus properties: single-stranded, negative-sense RNA, enveloped

INFECTIONS
PRIMARY
Measles, also called rubeola
Systemic: constitutional symptoms—cough, coryza, conjunctivitis, and photophobia; Koplik's spots (1)—most often on buccal mucosa
Skin: maculopapular rash (2)—begins at head spreads to extremities

OTHER
Complications:
  Nervous: subacute sclerosing panencephalitis (SSPE)
  Ear: otitis media
  Respiratory: pneumonia

EPIDEMIOLOGY
Transmission: respiratory droplets
High risk: unvaccinated individuals

DIAGNOSIS
Viral culture: measles infected cells are enlarged and contain multiple nuclei
Serology: antibody testing
PCR

PREVENTION
Vaccine: live, attenuated vaccine

TREATMENT
Supportive; vitamin A and immune globulin may reduce severity and prevent delayed recovery

Explanation: Measles is part of the Paramyxovirus family (like ● 31, Parainfluenza virus ●, ● 32, Respiratory syncytial virus (RSV) ●, and ● 19, Mumps virus ●), and is a single-stranded, negative-sense RNA virus. Measles begins with a prodrome phase (the 3 C's: cough, coryza, and conjunctivitis). This lasts about 2 to 3 days. Koplik's spots, which last 12 to 72 hours, may be present on the buccal mucosa. This is followed by the maculopapular exanthem, as described in this case.

Vignette: An otherwise healthy 11-year-old boy visits his pediatrician for a routine well-child examination. The child's vital signs are normal. On physical exam, three small flesh-colored and dome-shaped papules are noted on his trunk. The papules are clumped together and are depressed in the center. The exam is otherwise unremarkable. The boy states the papules appeared a couple of weeks ago and are painless. He thought they were warts, so he did not notify his parents. All routine laboratory tests are within normal limits.

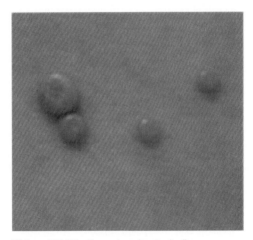

(1) *Source:* CDC (https://www.cdc.gov/poxvirus/molluscum-contagiosum/images/index-image.jpg)

DESCRIPTION

Taxonomy: Poxvirus family; *Molluscipoxvirus* genus
See also ● Variola virus ●
Virus properties: double-stranded DNA, enveloped

INFECTIONS
PRIMARY

Molluscum contagiosum
Skin: exanthem (1)—dome-shaped papules with central umbilication; often described as waxy; may be located anywhere on body excluding the palms and soles

PATHOGENESIS

Infects then replicates in epithelial cells.

EPIDEMIOLOGY

Transmission:
    Direct contact with exanthem
    Fomites
    Sexual contact
Associated with contact sports, such as wrestling
Mainly seen in children
High risk: individuals with HIV may have more serious infection

DIAGNOSIS

Usually made on clinical findings
Microscopy: identification of molluscum bodies, which are intracytoplasmic inclusions in epithelial cells, from infected tissue

TREATMENT

Immunocompetent—supportive

Explanation: Molluscum contagiosum is a self-limiting infection caused by a poxvirus. Small dome-shaped papules are present on the face, trunk, and extremities. This infection is often seen in children and is transmitted via direct contact with the papules or via fomites. Sexual transmission may occur as well, and in these cases papules may be noted in the genitalia or groin. In HIV patients, especially those with low CD4 counts, molluscum contagiosum may be more serious. Often papules are noted on the face in these cases. Another notable member of the poxvirus family is variola virus, the agent of smallpox. However, variola is part of the *Orthopoxvirus* genus, whereas molluscum contagiosum is part of the *Molluscipoxvirus* genus.

Vignette: A 4-year-old girl from rural Pakistan has a rash that is vesicular in appearance. Vesicles are present on the oral mucosa as well as on the face, trunk, and extremities, including her soles and palms. All the vesicles look similar in appearance. She has never been vaccinated.

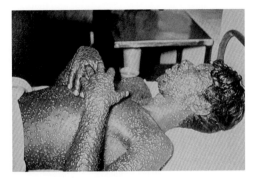

(1) *Source:* CDC/NIP/Barbara Rice
    CDC public health library PHIL (phil.cdc.gov) image No. 131
    (http://phil.cdc.gov/phil/details_linked.asp?pid=131)

DESCRIPTION

Taxonomy: Poxvirus family; *Orthopoxvirus* genus
See also ● 115, Molluscum contagiosum virus ●
Description: double-stranded DNA, enveloped

INFECTIONS
PRIMARY

Skin: smallpox—several forms: ordinary, vaccine modified, flat, and hemorrhagic
Ordinary: most common—macular, papular rash that develops into vesicles and pustules that crust; all lesions are in the same stage of development (1)

EPIDEMIOLOGY

Transmission:
Respiratory droplets
Contact with vesicle fluid, body fluid
Fomites

DIAGNOSIS

Electron microscopy
PCR

PREVENTION

Vaccine: live, attenuated vaccine

TREATMENT

Supportive

Explanation: This child has smallpox, caused by the variola virus. The rash is vesicular and centrifugally distributed, and there are often more vesicles on the face and oral mucosa than on the trunk. Fever and other nonspecific constitutional symptoms may precede the exanthem. This virus is spread by respiratory droplets, vesicular fluids, body fluids from infected individuals, and fomites. An important characteristic is that the vesicles are all in the same stages of development, which is a key difference from chickenpox (● 117, Varicella-zoster virus ●).

Micro gem: In chickenpox (VZV) the vesicles are all in different stages of development. In contrast, in ● 116, Smallpox virus (Variola virus) ● the vesicles are all in the same stage of development.

Vignette: A 4-year-old girl has a rash that is vesicular in appearance and itchy. The rash started on her neck, and she now has multiple vesicles on her stomach and back. Some of the vesicles are now crusting over, but some of the vesicles are still developing. She has not received her routine childhood vaccines.

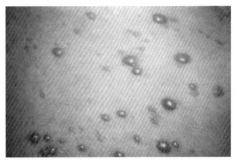

(1) *Source:* CDC/K.L. Hermann
CDC public health library PHIL (phil.cdc.gov) image No. 5407
(http://phil.cdc.gov/phil/details_linked.asp?pid=5407)

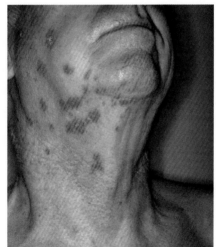

(2) *Source:* CDC/National Institute of Allergy and Infectious Diseases (NIAID)
CDC public health library PHIL (phil.cdc.gov) image No. 18254
(http://phil.cdc.gov/phil/details_linked.asp?pid=18254)

DESCRIPTION

Taxonomy: Herpesvirus family
See also ●48, Cytomegalovirus (CVM)●; ●51, Epstein-Barr virus (EBV)●; ●139, Herpes simplex virus (HSV)-1 and -2●; ●52, Human herpes virus-6 (HHV-6)●
Virus properties: double-stranded DNA, enveloped
Also called human herpes virus-3

INFECTIONS

PRIMARY

Varicella
Skin: varicella (i.e., chickenpox)—papules that turn into vesicles and pustules that crust (1); pruritic and all in different stages of development; starts on face and moves to extremities
Complications:
Skin: secondary bacterial skin infection
Nervous: encephalitis
Respiratory: pneumonia
Zoster
Skin: papules that develop into vesicles or bullae—usually limited to one dermatome (2). Pain, itching, or tingling may precede rash in same location
Nervous: neuritis
Complications
Skin: secondary bacterial skin infection
Head and neck: eye—keratitis
Nervous: meningitis

OTHER

Congenital
Skin: skin lesions
Head and neck: eye—ocular defects
Nervous: CNS abnormalities
TORCH = congenital infections
●14, *Toxoplasma gondii*●; **O**ther (●106, *Treponema pallidum*●, Varicella-zoster virus ●55, Parvovirus B19●); ●142, **R**ubella

virus●; ●48, **C**ytomegalovirus (CMV)●; ●139, **H**erpes simplex virus (HSV)-1 and -2●

PATHOGENESIS

After initial infection with varicella, virus establishes latency in sensory ganglia; reactivation results in zoster

EPIDEMIOLOGY

Transmission:
Respiratory droplets
Direct contact with vesicle fluid
Vertical: usually *in utero*—patients with an active VZV rash are advised to avoid contact with pregnant, unvaccinated women
Note: an unimmunized/not immune individual who comes in contact with shingles rash is at risk for contracting chickenpox, but not shingles.

DIAGNOSIS

Viral culture
Serology: antibody testing
Microscopy: Tzanck smear—cells from base of lesion are enlarged and multinucleated
PCR

PREVENTION

Vaccine
Varicella: live, attenuated vaccine
Zoster: live, attenuated vaccine; administered starting at age 60

TREATMENT

Varicella: supportive
Zoster: depends on immune status of host; acyclovir, valacyclovir, famciclovir

Explanation: This child has chickenpox, caused by the varicella virus. A typical rash is vesicular and is itchy, as described in this case. Fever and other nonspecific constitutional symptoms may precede the exanthem. This virus is spread by respiratory droplets, and the vesicular fluid is also contagious. An important characteristic is that the vesicles are all in different stages of development, which is a key difference from smallpox.

Vignette: An otherwise healthy 40-year-old man visits his physician for a pre-employment physical. He mentions that his feet have been abnormally dry and itchy. The bottom area of both feet is scaly and the surrounding skin is peeling. A KOH preparation from the skin shows the presence of hyphal elements.

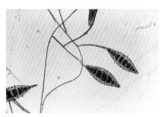

(1) *Source:* CDC/Dr. Lucille K. Georg
CDC public health library PHIL (phil.cdc.gov)
image No. 15472
(http://phil.cdc.gov/phil/details_linked.
asp?pid=15472)

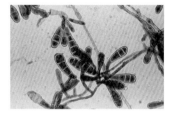

(2) *Source:* CDC/Dr. Lucille K. Georg
CDC public health library PHIL (phil.cdc.gov)
image No. 14588
(http://phil.cdc.gov/phil/details_linked.
asp?pid=14588)

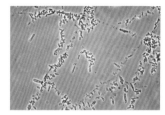

(3) *Source:* CDC/Dr. Libero Ajello
CDC public health library PHIL (phil.cdc.gov)
image No. 11006
(http://phil.cdc.gov/phil/details_linked.
asp?pid=11006)

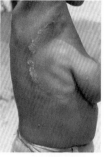

(4) *Source:* CDC/Dr. Lucille K. Georg
CDC public health library PHIL (phil.cdc.gov)
image No. 2909
(http://phil.cdc.gov/phil/details_linked.
asp?pid=2909)

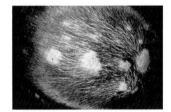

(5) *Source:* CDC/Dr. Lucille K. Georg
CDC public health library PHIL (phil.cdc.gov)
image No. 12546
(http://phil.cdc.gov/phil/details_linked.
asp?pid=12546)

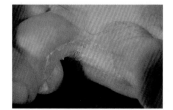

(6) *Source:* CDC/Dr. Lucille K. Georg
CDC public health library PHIL (phil.cdc.gov)
image No. 2939
(http://phil.cdc.gov/phil/details_linked.
asp?pid=2939)

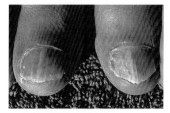

(7) *Source:* CDC/Dr. Edwin P. Ewing, Jr.
CDC public health library PHIL (phil.cdc.gov)
image No. 579
(http://phil.cdc.gov/phil/details_linked.
asp?pid=579)

DESCRIPTION Mold
Clinically significant morphological forms: macroconidia, microconidia

INFECTIONS
PRIMARY
Dermatophytosis also called cutaneous mycosis
Superficial infections of skin, hair, nails:
  Microsporum (1): infects skin and hair, rarely nails
  Epidermophyton (2): infects skin and nails, not hair
  Trichophyton (3): infects skin, hair, and nails
Glabrous skin: tinea corporis—often referred to as ringworm (4)
Hair/scalp: tinea capitis (5)
Nails: tinea unguium—also called onychomycosis (6)
Feet: tinea pedis—also called athlete's foot (7)
Groin: tinea cruris—also called jock itch
Note: this is not a complete list of "tinea" infections

EPIDEMIOLOGY Transmission:
  Direct contact with infected humans, animals, or soil
  Fomites

DIAGNOSIS Fungal culture
Microscopy: direct exam of specimen and identification of conidia or hyphae with KOH
Wood's lamp (black light/UV light): skin infected with *Microsporum* will fluoresce apple-green

TREATMENT Topical antifungals such as terbinafine and butenafine
Note: nyastatin is not effective against dermatophytes
Avoid use of antifungal/corticosteroid combinations

Explanation: Dermatophytes such as *Microsporum, Epidermophyton,* and *Trichophyton* are agents of superficial fungal infections and are most often not serious. This patient has tinea pedis, which is commonly referred to as athlete's foot. KOH preparations are useful for examining clinical specimens, as cellular debris and other background material is dissolved, allowing for better visualization of fungal organisms.

Vignette: An 18-year-old Caucasian man from Texas visits a physician in August because he hurt his back at work. He works in construction, and mostly outdoors. His history is otherwise unremarkable. His vital signs are normal, and during his physical exam patchy areas of hyperpigmentation are noted on his back, shoulders, and trunk. When viewed with a Wood's lamp, the areas of hyperpigmentation fluoresce yellow.

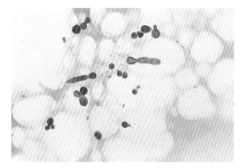

(1) *Source:* CDC/Dr. Lucille K. Georg
CDC public health library PHIL (phil.cdc.gov) image No. 3938
(http://phil.cdc.gov/phil/details_linked.asp?pid=3938)

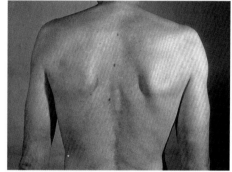

(2) *Source:* CDC/Dr. Lucille K. Georg
CDC public health library PHIL (phil.cdc.gov) image No. 12534
(http://phil.cdc.gov/phil/details_linked.asp?pid=12534)

DESCRIPTION
Yeast and hyphae
Yeast: budding yeast—"bowling ball" appearance (1)
Hyphae: vary in length
Yeast cells may cluster together and may be found with the hyphae giving a "spaghetti (hyphae)-and-meatball (yeast)" appearance

INFECTIONS

PRIMARY
Superficial infections of skin and hair: pityriasis versicolor (also called tinea versicolor)—hyperpigmented or hypopigmented patchy skin (2), seborrheic dermatitis, dandruff

OTHER
Systemic: fungemia

EPIDEMIOLOGY
Normal microbiota of skin
Transmission: overgrowth of normal microbiota
Transmission enhanced by heat and humidity, sweat, oily skin
High risk: fungemia associated with catheters in individuals on parenteral lipids, especially neonates

DIAGNOSIS
Fungal culture: requires long chain fatty acid— olive oil added to agar plate to aid growth
Microscopy: identification of characteristic yeast and hyphae
Wood's lamp (black light/UV light): skin infected with *M. furfur* will fluoresce orange-yellow

TREATMENT
Ketaconazole shampoo, selenium sulfide shampoo

Explanation: Pityriasis is a superficial infection of the skin caused by the yeast *Malassezia*. This pathogen is generally a commensal organism and not a common agent of infection. In pityriasis, skin may be hyperpigmented or hypopigmented. Excessive sweat and heat may enhance the growth of this organism. *Malassezia* fluoresces yellow or orange with a Wood's lamp.

Micro gem: *Sporothrix schenckii* is a thermally dimorphic fungus. Other thermally dimorphic fungi include ● 35, *Blastomyces dermatitidis* ●, ● 36, *Coccidioides immitis* and *posadasii* ●, ● 37, *Histoplasma capsulatum* ●, and ● 38, *Paracoccidiodes brasiliensis* ●.

Vignette: A 56-year-old woman presents with multiple wounds on her forearm. She has a history of injury to her hand while trimming the bushes in her yard. She states that initially she had one small pimple on her hand, and eventually several nodule-like lesions appeared on her arm. She is concerned because it is summer and she is embarrassed to have her arms uncovered. She is otherwise feeling well. Her vital signs are normal. On exam, four shallow ulcers are noted along the lymphatic channel, and a small amount of clear drainage is present. Her physical exam is otherwise unremarkable. The drainage from the ulcer shows yeast cells with elongated daughter yeast budding from the mother cell.

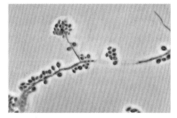

(1) *Source:* CDC/Dr. Libero Ajello
    CDC public health library PHIL (phil.cdc.gov)
    image No. 4220
    (http://phil.cdc.gov/phil/details_linked.
    asp?pid=4220)

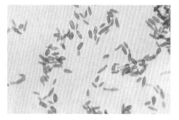

(2) *Source:* CDC/Dr. Lucille K. Georg
    CDC public health library PHIL (phil.cdc.gov)
    image No. 3944
    (http://phil.cdc.gov/phil/details_linked.
    asp?pid=3944)

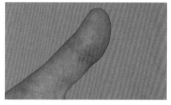

(3) *Source:* CDC/Dr. William Kaplan
    CDC public health library PHIL (phil.cdc.gov)
    image No. 3011
    (http://phil.cdc.gov/phil/details_linked.
    asp?pid=3011)

(4) *Source:* CDC/Dr. Lucille K. Georg
    CDC public health library PHIL (phil.cdc.gov)
    image No. 3940
    (http://phil.cdc.gov/phil/details_linked.
    asp?pid=3940)

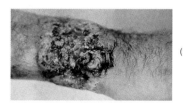

(5) *Source:* CDC/Dr. Lucille K. Georg
    CDC public health library PHIL (phil.cdc.gov)
    image No. 14547
    (http://phil.cdc.gov/phil/details_linked.
    asp?pid=14547)

DESCRIPTION Thermally dimorphic—exists as a mold at room temperature a yeast at body temperature

25°C: mold with thin hyphae and rosette-like conidia (1)

37°C: budding yeast; budding cells may be elongated, giving a "cigar body" appearance (2)

INFECTIONS Sporotrichosis

PRIMARY Skin and soft tissue/lymphatic:

Lymphocutaneous sporotrichosis: papule at site of infection (3) that ulcerates with nonpurulent drainage (4,5); lesions spread along the lymphatic channel

OTHER Respiratory: cavitary lesions, possible pulmonary infiltrates

Musculoskeletal: osteoarticular infections, osteomyelitis

Nervous: meningitis

EPIDEMIOLOGY Normal inhabitant of soil and various plants

Transmission:

Most infections: traumatic penetration of conidia into skin or subcutaneous tissue

Respiratory: inhalation of conidia

Often referred to as rose gardener's disease—high risk of contracting infection following a thorn prick

DIAGNOSIS Fungal culture

Microscopy: identification of budding "cigar body"–like yeast from tissue

TREATMENT Depends on infection type

Lymphocutaneous: itraconazole

Pulmonary: amphotericin B

Explanation: This patient has lymphocutaneous sporotrichosis, which is caused by the dimorphic fungus *Sporothrix schenckii*. The pathogen enters the skin following trauma. The hallmark of infection is a primary lesion at the point of entry and secondary lesions along the lymphatic channel. Usually the individual is otherwise well, and very few systemic manifestations are seen. It is important to note that other pathogens, such as ● 28, *Nocardia* ●, ● 132, Nontuberculosis *Mycobacterium* ● (*Mycobacterium marinum*), and ● 111, *Francisella tularensis* ●, may also present with similar manifestations. Culture and microscopic evaluation is the best mechanism of identifying this pathogen.

Micro gem: *Leishmania*, ● 37, *Histoplasma capsulatum* ●, and ● 103, *Klebsiella granulomatis* ● can be found within histocytes.

Vignette: A 37-year-old man notices a small pimple on his arm. Within a week the pimple has developed into a larger ulcer with a central depression. A small amount of yellowish drainage surrounds the ulcer. The man has a recent history of travel to India. A skin biopsy specimen stained with Giemsa demonstrates the presence of an oval-shaped amastigote within macrophages.

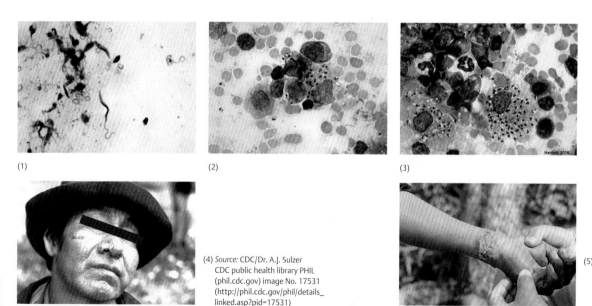

(1)

(2)

(3)

(4) *Source:* CDC/Dr. A.J. Sulzer
CDC public health library PHIL
(phil.cdc.gov) image No. 17531
(http://phil.cdc.gov/phil/details_
linked.asp?pid=17531)

(5) *Source:* CDC/Dr. A.J. Sulzer
CDC public health library PHIL
(phil.cdc.gov) image No. 14971
(http://phil.cdc.gov/phil/details_
linked.asp?pid=14971)

121 *Leishmania*

DESCRIPTION

Protozoa: flagellate
Clinically significant morphological forms:
Promastigote—flagellated form found in sandfly (1)
Amastigote (2,3)—non-flagellated form found in humans
Subgenera: *L. leishmania* (LL), *L. viannia* (LV)
Clinically significant species include (not a complete list):
Old World species: *L.L donovani, L.L infantum, L.L. major, L.L. tropica*,
New World species: *L.V. braziliensis, L. mexicana*

INFECTIONS
PRIMARY

Infections may also be classified as Old World and New World
Old World
L.L. donovani, L.L. infantum
Systemic: visceral leishmaniasis (VL) also called dumdum fever and kala-azar—indolent infection with intermittent fever, weight loss, malaise, abdominal pain, hepatospleno-megaly, and pancytopenia
Skin: post-VL skin lesions—papules or macules that may form nodules following treatment for VL
L.L. major, L.L., tropica, L. mexicana (and others species)
Skin: cutaneous leishmaniasis (most common) (4,5)—papule that develops into ulcer at bite site
New World
L.V. braziliensis
Skin and soft tissue/other: mucosal or mucocutaneous leish-maniasis (rare)—lesions that destroy mucous membranes

PATHOGENESIS

Obligate intracellular pathogen—invades macrophages

EPIDEMIOLOGY

Transmission: bite of a sandfly
Geographic distribution: species specific, but mostly seen in tropical climates
Old World species: mainly seen in Middle East, Mediterra-nean, North Africa and South East Europe
New World species: South and Central America

DIAGNOSIS

Microscopy: identification of amastigotes in macrophages of spleen, liver, and bone marrow
PCR
Serology: antibody testing

TREATMENT

Depends on species, infection type and severity, and immune status
Visceral leishmaniasis: liposomal amphotericin B
Cutaneous leishmaniasis: sodium sibogluconate

Explanation: This man has cutaneous leishmaniasis caused by the protozoan par-asite *Leishmania*. There are several species of *Leishmania* that have been implicated in cutaneous leishmaniasis, and different species may be localized to different geo-graphic areas. More serious forms of leishmaniasis include mucocutaneous infec-tions and visceral leishmaniasis. *Leishmania* is an intracellular parasite that lives within macrophages. The amastigote form can be seen within macrophages, which aids in diagnosis.

Vignette: A 28-year-old woman presents with a 2-week history of a rash and diarrhea. The rash is not itchy, and she denies blood in her stool. She also reports she has been feeling extremely tired for the past month. About 2 months ago, she returned from an African safari trip to Kenya and Tanzania, during which she had gone camping near Lake Mara and had waterskied. Her vital signs are normal. Several small papules and macules are noted on her trunk on physical exam. A CBC shows eosinophilia. A stool specimen demonstrates the presence of several oval-shaped parasite eggs.

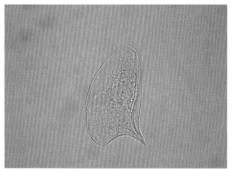

(1)

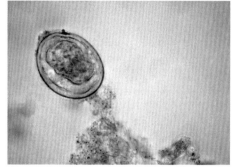

(2)

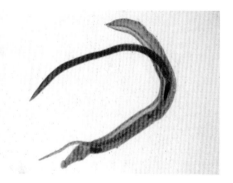

(3) Male and female adult worms in copulation.

DESCRIPTION

Platyhelminth / flatworm: trematode / fluke
Clinically significant morphological forms: ova (eggs) (1,2); adults (3)

INFECTIONS

PRIMARY

Acute schistosomiasis
Gastrointestinal diarrhea, abdominal pain
Systemic: Katayama fever

LIFE CYCLE

Ova released in fresh water from human stool; develop into miracidia; miracidia penetrate snails; miracidia mature to larvae in snails; snails release cercariae; cercaria penetrate human skin; enter circulation and migrate to hepatic portal system; mature into adults (3); adults migrate and live in mesenteric plexus of small and large intestine

EPIDEMIOLOGY

Transmission: contact with contaminated fresh water
Geographic distribution
S. mansoni: mainly seen in Africa and South America
S. japonicum: mainly seen in East Asia

DIAGNOSIS

Microscopy: identification of ova in stool or tissue; *S. mansoni—*large lateral spine (1); *S. japonicum—*small, short, knob-like lateral spine (2)
Serology: antibody testing
CBC: eosinophilia

TREATMENT

Praziquantel

Explanation: Acute schistosomiasis or Katayama fever is caused by several species of schistosomes, including *S. mansoni and S. japonicum*. *S. mansoni* is mainly seen in Africa, whereas *S. japonicum* is mainly found in East Asia. Humans are infected following skin penetration of the larvae, which are found in fresh water. Manifestations of Katayama fever include urticaria, fever, cough, abdominal pain, and diarrhea.

Vignette: A 47-year-old man presents with muscle pain and weakness, fever, headache, and swelling in the face. He reports that he recently also experienced diarrhea. He denies blood in the stool. About 1 month prior, he had traveled to Germany, where he toured a sausage factory and consumed samples of beef and pork sausage. On exam, his temperature is 39.1°C (102.4°F), and significant facial edema is noted, predominantly around his eyelids. The CBC demonstrates elevated eosinophils. Stool culture is normal, and a stool O&P test is negative.

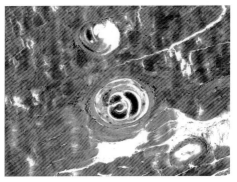
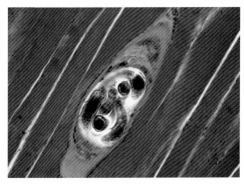

(1) (2)

DESCRIPTION Nemathelminth / roundworms
Clinically significant morphological forms: ova (eggs), larvae (1), adult worms

INFECTIONS

PRIMARY Trichinosis
  Gastrointestinal: initial phase—mainly asymptomatic; nausea, vomiting, and diarrhea
  Musculoskeletal: later phase—generalized muscle pain, tenderness, swelling, and weakness; periorbital edema

OTHER Cardiovascular: myocarditis (due to inflammatory response and not pathogen presence)
Nervous: meningitis, encephalitis

LIFE CYCLE Ingestion of encysted larvae; larvae excyst in stomach and invade small intestine mucosa; mature into adults; adults lay eggs, which mature to larvae; larvae are deposited in mucosa and travel via circulation to skeletal muscle and encyst

EPIDEMIOLOGY Transmission: ingestion of encysted larva—commonly associated with undercooked pork and bear meat

DIAGNOSIS Serology: antibody testing
Microscopy: identification of larva from skeletal muscle (within nurse cell) (2)
CBC: eosinophilia

TREATMENT Mild cases: supportive—usually self-limiting
Severe cases: albendazole

Explanation: Trichinosis is caused by the nematode *Trichinella spiralis*. The pathogen is most often transmitted via ingestion of undercooked pork. Initial diarrhea and other symptoms such as nausea and vomiting are due to the intestinal invasion of the larva. The pathogen then encysts in skeletal muscle, leading to myalgia, weakness, headache, and periorbital edema. Eosinophilia is often present after the worm leaves the intestine. After the worm leaves the intestine, stool O&P results may be negative, but the larvae may be observed encysted within skeletal muscle.

124 *Bacteroides*

Micro gem: *Bacteroides fragilis* is the most commonly recovered clinical anaerobic pathogen. Other frequently isolated anaerobes are listed in the table in the appendix.

Vignette: A 48-year-old man presents with a 3-day history of abdominal pain and bloating, and fever. His history is significant for an appendectomy approximately 3 weeks prior to the onset of symptoms. His temperature is 38.8°C (101.8°F), and his heart rate is 130 bpm. A CBC shows elevated WBCs. A CT scan shows fluid collection with air bubbles, suggestive of an abscess. After 2 days, blood cultures grow gram-negative bacilli in the anaerobic bottles but not the aerobic bottles.

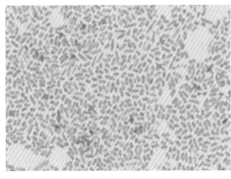

(1)

DESCRIPTION
Gram-negative rod or coccobacilli (1)
Obligate anaerobe
Most clinically significant pathogens are in the *Bacteroides fragilis* (BF) group—main clinically significant species is *B. fragilis*

INFECTIONS

PRIMARY
May affect any anatomic site
Gastrointestinal: intra-abdominal abscesses, peritonitis
Systemic: bacteremia
Reproductive: gynecologic abscesses—associated with intra-uterine devices

OTHER
Gastrointestinal: watery diarrhea
Head and neck: abscesses
Nervous system: abscesses
Skin and soft tissue: abscesses

PATHOGENESIS
Capsule
Enterotoxin

EPIDEMIOLOGY
Normal microbiota of mucosal surfaces, mainly of GI tract
Transmission: mostly from endogenous strains due to perforation of local anatomic site
High risk: peritonitis—ruptured appendix, ischemic bowel, ruptured diverticulitis, other abdominal surgical procedures

DIAGNOSIS
Culture

TREATMENT
Metronidazole, piperacillin-tazobactam
Resistant to penicillin due to production of beta-lactamases

Explanation: Anaerobic organisms, especially *Bacteroides fragilis*, are frequently implicated in intra-abdominal abscesses. Often, intra-abdominal abscesses are polymicrobial. *B. fragilis* is an anaerobic gram-negative bacillus. The presence of gram-negative bacilli in the blood cultures suggests intra-abdominal sepsis, which in turn suggests the presence of an intra-abdominal abscess. The CT results confirm these findings.

Vignette: A 45-year-old man presents with a one-week history of headache, fever, and muscle aches. He has a recent history of camping in a wooded area in upstate New York. His vitals are normal and physical exam reveals an erythematous rash with a central clearing on his upper back. He denies pain or pruitis. Serological tests confirm the identity of the pathogen responsible for this infection.

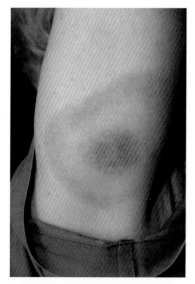

(1) *Source:* CDC/ James Gathany
CDC public health library PHIL (phil.cdc.gov) Image #9875
http://phil.cdc.gov/phil/details_linked.asp?pid=9875

DESCRIPTION
Spirochete
Gram-negative cell wall—has outer membrane and LPS
Does not Gram stain well

INFECTIONS
PRIMARY
Lyme Disease
Multi-system
Stage 1
    Skin and soft tissue: rash—erythema migrans (target-shaped/bulls eye shaped) (1)
    Systemic: constitutional symptoms
Stage 2
    Cardiovascular: AV nodal block
    Nervous: meningitis, Bell's palsy
    Musculoskeletal: transient arthritis
    Skin and soft tissue: skin lesions
Stage 3
    Musculoskeletal: chronic arthritis

EPIDEMIOLOGY
Transmission: bite of a tick (*Ixodes scapularis*)
    See also ● 56, *Babesia microti* ●
Geographic distribution: in U.S. higher incidence in Northeast, Midwest, and Northern California

DIAGNOSIS
Serology: antibody testing
PCR

TREATMENT
Depends on stage and infection site
    Early infections: doxycycline, amoxicillin
    Nervous system infections: ceftriaxone

Explanation: Lyme disease is caused by the spirochete *Borrelia burgdorferi*. Classic manifestations include erythema migrans as described in this case. This pathogen may be seen many parts of the country but there is a higher incidence in areas of the Northeast such as Connecticut and upstate New York.

Micro gem: All staphylococci are catalase positive. In contrast, all streptococci are catalase negative.

Vignette: A 67-year-old man presents with a 2-day history of dyspnea and syncope. His history is significant for a mitral valve replacement approximately 30 days prior to the onset of his current symptoms. Physical examination demonstrates a systolic murmur. Echocardiography shows vegetations on the mitral valve. Blood cultures are positive and grow coagulase-negative, gram-positive cocci in clusters.

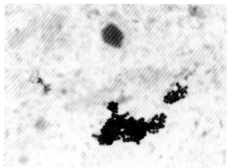

(1)

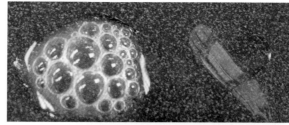

(2) Left, catalase positive.
Right, catalase negative.

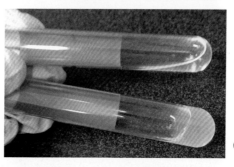

(3) Top, coagulase negative.
Bottom, coagulase positive.

DESCRIPTION
Gram-positive cocci in clusters (1)
Many clinically significant species including: *S. epidermidis, S. lugdunensis,* ● 98, *Staphylococcus saprophyticus* ●

INFECTIONS
PRIMARY

Cardiovascular: *S. epidermidis, S. lugdunensis*—infective endocarditis—native and prosthetic valve
Nervous system: meningitis, shunt infections
Systemic: bacteremia
Skin and soft tissue, musculoskeletal: *S. epidermidis*—surgical site infections, prosthetic joint infections
Renal/urinary: *S. saprophyticus, S. epidermidis*— UTIs

PATHOGENESIS
Biofilm formation—forms biofilms on plastic devices such as intravascular or urinary catheters. Bacteria from the biofilm can then seed the bloodstream or urinary tract, resulting in infection.

EPIDEMIOLOGY
Normal microbiota of the skin
Transmission: most often displacement of endogenous strains
S. epidermidis is the most common cause of prosthetic valve endocarditis within one year of placement
High risk:
 Endocarditis: cardiac device or prosthetic valve
 Nervous system: ventriculoperitoneal (VP) shunt or other device
 Bacteremia: intravascular catheter
 Joint infections: prosthetic joint or other hardware
 UTI: indwelling urinary catheter

DIAGNOSIS
Culture: catalase positive (2), coagulase negative (3)

TREATMENT
Methicillin susceptible—oxacillin, nafcillin, cefazolin
Methicillin resistant—vancomycin, daptomycin, linezolid

Explanation: In infectious endocarditis, native or prosthetic valves may be infected with coagulase-negative staphylococci. All staphylococci are catalase positive. Only *S. aureus* is coagulase positive. All other staphylococci, other than ● 134, *Staphylococcus aureus* ●, are classified in the broad category of coagulase-negative staphylococci.

Vignette: A previously healthy 39-year-old woman presents with fever, headache, chills, sweats, myalgia, and a dry, nonproductive cough of 1-week duration. She states the symptoms occurred abruptly. She works as a veterinarian at a farm, and she has not traveled outside of the United States recently. Her temperature is 40.2°C (104.4°F). Her physical examination reveals inspiratory crackles. Her peripheral WBC count is normal. Serological testing demonstrates the presents of *Coxiella burnetii* antibodies.

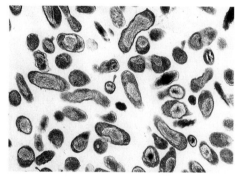

(1) *Source:* CDC/National Institute of Allergy and Infectious
Diseases (NIAID); Rocky Mountain Laboratories, NIH
CDC public health library PHIL (phil.cdc.gov) image No. 8158
(http://phil.cdc.gov/phil/details_linked.asp?pid=18158)

DESCRIPTION Gram-negative cell wall; coccobacilli shape (1), very tiny

INFECTIONS
PRIMARY
Q fever
May be asymptomatic
    Acute
        Systemic: febrile flu-like illness
        Respiratory: pneumonia—typically starts as atypical pneumonia
        Liver: hepatitis
    Chronic
        Cardiovascular: infective endocarditis

PATHOGENESIS
Antigen variation
Spore-like form of the organism enables it to survive in environment
Obligate intracellular pathogen—lives within macrophages

EPIDEMIOLOGY
Transmission:
    Inhalation of aerosols from contaminated animal secretions including urine, feces, milk, placenta—commonly associated animals include goats, sheep
    Foodborne (rare): ingestion of milk from infected animal
High risk: veterinarians, farmers

DIAGNOSIS Serology: antibody testing—titers of acute and convalescent sera
PCR

TREATMENT Doxycycline

Explanation: *Coxiella burnetii* is the agent of Q fever. The most common manifestations of acute infections are nonspecific febrile illness, pneumonia, and hepatitis. The pathogen is transmitted via aerosols from contaminated secretions from infected animals, especially farm animals such as goats and sheep. Veterinarians, such as the patient in this case, are at high risk for infections. *C. burnetii* has a gram-negative cell wall, but are tiny; hence, Gram stain may not be the best mechanism of diagnosis.

Vignette: An 81-year-old man who lives in a nursing home is transferred to the hospital with fever and chills. The nurse notes that his Foley catheter bag contains cloudy urine. On examination, his temperature is 39.0°C (102.2°F). Urine from the catheter is collected for urinalysis, and the culture and grows > 100,000 CFUs of a gram-positive coccus in chains.

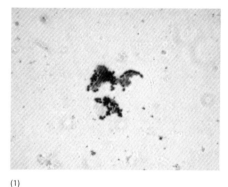

(1)

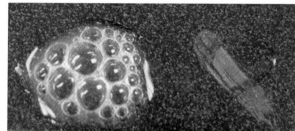

(2) Left, catalase positive.
    Right. catalase negative.

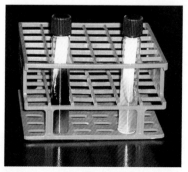

(3) Left, bile esculin positive.
    Right, bile esculin negative.

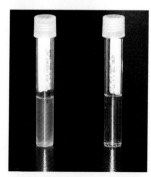

(4) Left, no growth in 6.5% NaCl.
    Right, growth in 6.5% NaCl.

DESCRIPTION
Gram-positive cocci often in pairs and short chains (1)
Common clinically significant species: *E. faecalis, E. faecium*

INFECTIONS
PRIMARY
Cardiovascular: infective endocarditis
Gastrointestinal: intra-abdominal and biliary tract abscesses
Renal/urinary: UTIs
Reproductive: pelvic abscess
Skin and soft tissue: wound infections
Systemic: bacteremia

PATHOGENESIS
Adhesins: tissue destruction—cytolysins and gelatinase
Vancomycin resistance—mediated by *vanA* and *vanB* genes (and less often *vanC* and *D*)
Isolates referred to as VRE—vancomycin resistant *Enterococcus*

EPIDEMIOLOGY
Colonizes the GI tract
Transmission: most often displacement of endogenous strains
Common nosocomial pathogen
Some individuals may colonize VRE in the GI tract. These individuals may then spread VRE within the hospital
High risk:
Hospitalization
Endocarditis: prosthetic heart valve
GI: intestinal surgery
Renal/urinary: indwelling urinary catheter
Skin and soft tissue: burns, diabetes

DIAGNOSIS
Culture: alpha, beta or gamma hemolytic, catalase negative (2), growth in bile (3), growth in high NaCl (6.5%) (4)

TREATMENT
Depends on species, infection type, and susceptibility to penicillin and vancomycin
For penicillin susceptible strains—penicillin
For VRE: daptomycin plus ampicillin, dalfopristin/quinupristin
Note: most strains of *E. faecium* are resistant to penicillin, aminoglycosides, and vancomycin

Explanation: *Enterococcus* is a common nosocomial pathogen and is frequently associated with catheter-related urinary tract infections. Enterococci are gram-positive cocci in chains, and vancomycin resistance is a significant nosocomial problem.

Vignette 1: A 34-year-old man visits his physician complaining of pain when urinating. His vital signs and physical examination are unremarkable. The urine is positive for leukocyte esterase and nitrites. His urine culture grows a lactose positive organism on MacConkey agar.

Vignette 2: A 2-day-old girl is brought to the emergency department with a fever. Her mother states that the infant has been crying and is inconsolable and refuses to eat. The infant was born at home, full-term, via a vaginal delivery. The baby's rectal temperature is 39.3°C (102.7°F), and on examination her fontanelle is full. A Gram stain from the CSF reveals gram-negative rods.

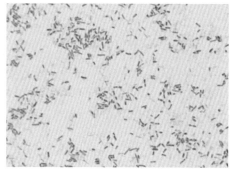

(1)

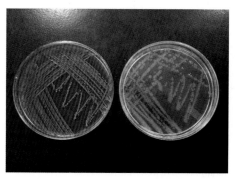

(2) MacConkey agar. Left, lactose positive. Right, lactose negative.

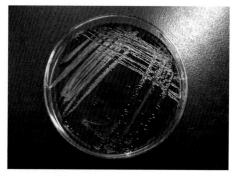

(3)

DESCRIPTION

Gram-negative rod (1); part of *Enterobacteriaceae* family
See also ●103, *Klebsiella granulomatis* ●; ●131, *Klebsiella pneumoniae* ●; ●97, *Proteus* ●; ●47, *Salmonella enterica* serotype typhi and paratyphi ●; ●70, Nontyphoidal *Salmonella* ●; ●71, *Shigella* ●; ●74, *Yersinia enterocolitica* and *pseudotuberculosis* ●; ●138, *Yersinia pestis* ●
Clinically important strains include:
Uropathogenic *Escherichia coli* (UPEC)
●64, Enteroaggregative *Escherichia coli* (EAEC) ●
●65, Enterohemorrhagic *Escherichia coli* (EHEC) ●, also called shiga toxin producing *E. coli* (STEC)
●66, Enteroinvasive *Escherichia coli* (EIEC) ●
●67, Enteropathogenic *Escherichia coli* (EPEC) ●
●68, Enterotoxigenic *Escherichia coli* (ETEC) ●

INFECTIONS

PRIMARY

Nervous: neonatal meningitis
Gastrointestinal: gastroenteritis
Renal/urinary: UTIs

OTHER

Biliary tract: ascending cholangitis
Respiratory: pneumonia
Skin and soft tissue: wound infections
Systemic: bacteremia

PATHOGENESIS

Meningitis: capsule—also called K1 antigen
UTI: pili/fimbriae
LPS—also called endotoxin; contributes to sepsis
Alpha-hemolysin
Adhesins
Gastroenteritis: enterotoxins
EHEC: shiga-like toxin/verotoxin—inhibits protein synthesis
ETEC: heat-labile (LT) toxin—increases cAMP and heat-stabile (ST) toxin—increases cGMP

EPIDEMIOLOGY

Some strains are normal microbiota of the GI tract; may also colonize vagina
Transmission: usually displacement of endogenous strains
Meningitis: vertical—usually perinatal
Gastroenteritis: foodborne, fecal-oral
Most common bacterial agent of UTIs

DIAGNOSIS

Culture: lactose positive– pink on MacConkey agar (2) and green metallic sheen on eosin methylene blue (EMB) agar (3); indole positive
EHEC only—sorbitol negative
Antigen detection for K1 strains

TREATMENT

Varies with infection site and clinical setting
Cephalosporins, ampicillin, piperacillin-tazobactam, aztreonam, trimethoprim-sulfamethoxazole, fosfomycin (for UTIs)
Frequent resistance:
Extended-spectrum beta-lactamase (ESBL) strains—resistant to cephalosporins—carbapenems are often effective in these cases
Carbapenemase producing strains—resistant to carbapenems—colistin (for UTIs) or polymyxin B plus meropenem may be effective in these cases

Explanation 1: *Escherichia coli*, a gram-negative rod, is one of the most common clinically recovered pathogens of urinary tract infections. MacConkey agar is selective for enteric gram-negative pathogens, and differential for lactose production. *E. coli* is lactose positive. One of the main virulence mechanisms of uropathogenic *E. coli* is P-fimbriae, which aids the organism in adhering to the bladder mucosa, forming a biofilm and establishing an infection.

Explanation 2: Several pathogens are implicated in neonatal meningitis. Common bacterial agents of neonatal meningitis include the gram-positive coccus ●5, *Streptococcus agalactiae* ● (group B streptococci), the gram-positive rod 3, ●*Listeria monocytogenes* ●, and the gram-negative rod *Escherichia coli*, K1. *E. coli* K1 has a capsule that aids the organism in evading the immune system and establishing more invasive infections, such as meningitis. *E. coli* strains, including the K1 strain, may colonize the vagina in healthy women and may be transmitted to babies during parturition.

Micro gem: Encapsulated strains are responsible for most invasive *H. influenzae* infections, including meningitis.

Vignette: A 4-year-old girl presents to the emergency department with difficulty swallowing and difficulty breathing, and fever. Her mother states that the symptoms had just begun earlier that day. At the time of examination, the girls' temperature is 40.1°C (104.2°F). On exam the girl appears visibly ill and respiratory distress and stridor are observed. Additionally, while seated she is leaning forward with her mouth opening and she is drooling. She has not been vaccinated.

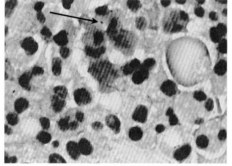

(1)

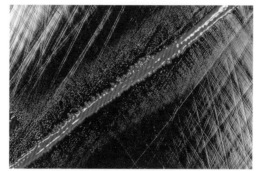

(3) *Source:* CDC/Dr. Mike Miller
CDC public health library PHIL (phil.cdc.gov) image No. 1047
(http://phil.cdc.gov/phil/details_linked.asp?pid=1047)

DESCRIPTION Gram-negative rod or coccobacilli (1)

INFECTIONS
PRIMARY

Invasive: *H. influenzae* type b (Hib) and other encapsulated strains
  Head and neck: epiglottis—epiglottitis
  Nervous: meningitis
  Respiratory: pneumonia
  Systemic: bacteremia
Noninvasive: mainly nontypeable (non-encapsulated) strains
  Head and neck:
    Ear—otitis media
    Eye—conjunctivitis
  Respiratory: sinusitis, pneumonia, acute exacerbation of COPD
    See also ● 16, *Moraxella catarrhalis* ●; ● 136, *Streptococcus pneumoniae* ●

PATHOGENESIS Capsule: types a to f; Hib capsule composed of polyribitol phosphate (PRP)
LPS, also called endotoxin—contributes to sepsis
IgA protease: destroys IgA
  See also ● 105, *Neisseria gonorrhoeae* ●; ● 4, *Neisseria meningitidis* ●; ● 136, *Streptococcus pneumoniae* ●

EPIDEMIOLOGY Nontypeable strains are normal respiratory microbiota.
Transmission of Hib: respiratory droplets or contact with respiratory secretions
Meningitis age distribution: mostly in children (but vaccination has decreased incidence)
High risk:
  Unvaccinated individuals

Asplenic individuals are at high risk for encapsulated *Haemophilus* since the spleen is important in the defense against encapsulated bacteria
  See also ● 136, *Streptococcus pneumoniae* ●; ● 4, *Neisseria meningitidis* ●

DIAGNOSIS Culture: best growth on chocolate agar; requires X (hemin) and V (*nicotinamide adenine dinucleotide* [NAD]) factors for growth provided by chocolate agar
  See also ● 102, *Haemophilus ducreyi* ●
Satellites around *S. aureus* on blood agar (2)
Requires 5 to 10% CO_2 for growth

PREVENTION Vaccine for Hib: conjugate vaccine (PRP conjugated to tetanus toxoid)

TREATMENT Life-threatening: cefotaxime, ceftriaxone
Non–life-threatening: amoxicillin-clavulanate, oral cephalosporins

ANIMATION http://go.thieme.com/microb/Video130.1

Explanation: The key features of epiglottis include difficulty breathing and swallowing, drooling and stridor. Infected individuals often assume the tripod position, in which they lean forward with their hands on their knees or another surface. The most common bacterial pathogen involved in epiglottitis is *Haemophilus influenzae*, especially *H. influenzae* type b. *H. influenzae* is a gram-negative coccobacillus, and infections may be prevented with vaccination. This organism needs both X factor (hemin) and V factor (NAD), to grow. Therefore, *H. influenzae* does not typically grow on blood agar, which only has X factor available, which is provided by either intact or lysed red blood cells. *H. influenzae* may however be found as satellite colonies or tiny colonies growing around ● 134, *Staphylococcus aureus* ● on blood agar. This is because *S. aureus* is beta-hemolytic and lyses the red blood cells in the blood agar, releasing the V factor which is an intracellular component of red blood cells.

Micro gem: *Klebsiella pneumoniae* and ●129, *Escherichia coli*● are the most common bacterial pathogens involved in ascending cholangitis.

Vignette: A 58-year-old homeless man presents to the emergency department with fever, chest pain, and cough productive of blood-tinged sputum. Upon examination the man is clearly intoxicated. He states he drinks whenever he can, but denies smoking cigarettes or using illicit drugs. His temperature is 38.9°C (102.0°F), and his respiratory rate is 29 breaths/minute. Decreased breath sounds and crackles in the right lower field are noted upon lung examination. His CBC demonstrates elevated WBCs. A chest radiograph reveals an infiltrate in the right lower lobe. A sputum culture demonstrates the presence of lactose-positive gram-negative rod.

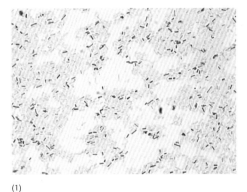

(1)

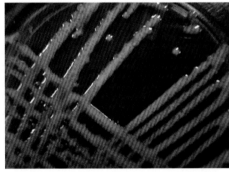

(2)

DESCRIPTION

Gram-negative rod (1); part of *Enterobacteriaceae* family
See also ● 129, *Escherichia coli* ●; ● 103, *Klebsiella granulomatis* ●; ● 97, *Proteus* ●; ● 47, *Salmonella enterica* serotype typhi and paratyphi ●; ● 70, Nontyphoidal *Salmonella* ●; ● 71, *Shigella* ●; ● 74, *Yersinia enterocolitica* and *pseudotuberculosis* ●; ● 138, *Yersinia pestis* ●

INFECTIONS

PRIMARY

Renal/urinary: UTIs, renal abscess
Respiratory: pneumonia, acute exacerbation of COPD, lung abscess
    Sputum is thick and blood-tinged ("currant jelly")
Systemic: bacteremia

OTHER

Biliary tract: ascending cholangitis
Cardiovascular: infective endocarditis
Liver: abscess
Nervous: meningitis, brain abscess
Skin and soft tissue: cellulitis, wound infections

PATHOGENESIS

Capsule: many capsular serotypes
Pili
LPS, also called endotoxin—contributes to sepsis

EPIDEMIOLOGY

Normal microbiota of the gastrointestinal tract
Transmission: endogenous strains or person-to-person either directly or via contaminated fomites, especially medical devices
Common nosocomial pathogen
High risk:
    Immunocompromised
    Diabetics
    Pneumonia—alcoholics at risk due to aspiration following emesis

DIAGNOSIS

Culture (2): lactose positive, mucoid colonies (due to the capsule)

TREATMENT

Agents vary with clinical setting and resistance
Cefazolin, ceftriaxone, piperacillin-tazobactam
Increasing resistance:
    Extended-spectrum beta-lactamase (ESBL) strains—resistant to cephalosporins—carbapenems are often effective in these cases
    Carbapenemase producing strains—resistant to carbapenems—colistin (for UTIs) or polymyxin B plus meropenem are often effective in these cases

Explanation: *Klebsiella pneumoniae* is a gram-negative rod that belongs to the *Enterobacteriaceae* family. This organism causes a variety of infections including wound, urinary tract, and respiratory infections. Respiratory infections may present as consolidation or "typical" pneumonia, such as in this case, and a key clue is the presence of blood-tinged sputum, often described as "currant-jelly" like. One of the main pathogenesis features of this organism is the presence of a capsule that causes this organism to appear mucoid on culture media.

Vignette: A 34-year-old woman presents with fever, fatigue, and weight loss. She has previously been diagnosed as HIV positive. She has lost 10 pounds over the past month. Her temperature is 38.8°C (101.8°F). She is ill appearing and pale. On examination, the liver edge is below the costal margin. Her CD4 count is 36 cells/mm^3. Blood cultures demonstrate the presence of acid-fast bacilli.

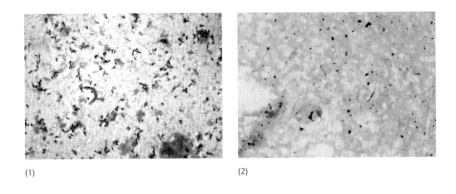

(1)

(2)

DESCRIPTION

Acid-fast bacilli (AFB) (1,2)
Mycolic acid (a type of fatty acid) in cell wall
Does not Gram stain
Includes several species:
Mycobacterium avium complex (MAC)—includes *M. avium* and *M. intracellulare*
M. kansasii
M. marinum
● 112, *M leprae* ●
Also referred to as *Mycobacterium* other than tuberculosis (MOTT)

INFECTIONS
PRIMARY

M. avium complex
Systemic: disseminated infection (fever, weight loss, night sweats)
Respiratory: pulmonary disease
M. kansasii
Respiratory: pulmonary infection, similar to TB
M. marinum
Skin and soft tissue: wound infections; granulomatous lesions; may spread along lymphatic channel

EPIDEMIOLOGY

Most nontuberculosis *Mycobacterium* are ubiquitous in the environment.
M. avium complex
Transmission: ingestion, inhalation—not transmitted person-to-person
Disseminated infection associated with AIDS and CD4 T cell < 50 cells/mm³
Pulmonary disease associated with elderly

M. kansasii
Transmission: ingestion, inhalation—not transmitted person-to-person
M. marinum
Transmission: penetration of skin following trauma
Associated with fish tanks, swimming pools, and water sources

DIAGNOSIS

Culture
Microscopy: acid-fast stains
Ziehl-Neelsen—"hot" stain (slides are heated while the primary stain is added)
Kinyoun—"cold" stain (heat is not necessary)
Acid-fast bacteria stain bright pink with Ziehl-Neelson and Kinyoun stains (1,2)
Auramine-rhodamine—fluorescent stain
Nucleic acid amplification

TREATMENT

Depends on species and immune status of host
Combination antimicrobial treatment may be used
Clarithromycin, azithromycin, ethambutol, rifampin

Explanation: Disseminated *Mycobacterium avium* complex (MAC) infections are seen mainly in immunocompromised individuals, especially in AIDS when the CD4 count is < 50 cells/mm³. Infections are often nonspecific and include the symptoms described in this case, as well as abdominal pain, diarrhea, and shortness of breath. This pathogen is most often recovered from blood and occasionally from bone marrow and is an acid-fast bacillus.

Micro gem: Pathogens with capsules include *Pseudomonas aeruginosa*, ●136, *Streptococcus pneumoniae* ●, ●131, *Klebsiella pneumoniae* ●, ●103, *Klebsiella granulomatis* ●, ●130, *Haemophilus influenzae* type b ●, ●4, *Neisseria meningitidis* ●, and ●11, *Cryptococcus neoformans* and *gatti* ●

Vignette 1: A 9-year-old boy presents to his pediatrician with an earache. He is on summer vacation and has spent many hours at the local community swimming pool. On examination, the physician notes that the boy's external ear is red and that there is greenish drainage coming from the ear. The drainage grows lactose-negative, gram-negative rod.

Vignette 2: A 54-year-old man has been in the hospital intensive care unit (ICU) on a ventilator for approximately 3 weeks as a result of a motor vehicle collision. The respiratory therapist notices that the patient's tracheal secretions are more purulent than before and notifies the physician, who orders a chest X-ray. The X-ray reveals diffuse bilateral infiltrates. A bronchoscopy is performed, and the aspirate is sent to the microbiology laboratory for Gram stain and bacterial culture. The Gram stain of the aspirate demonstrates an oxidase-positive, gram-negative rod.

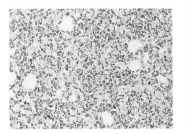

(1)

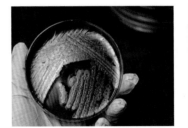

(2) MacConkey agar. Left, lactose positive. Right, lactose negative.

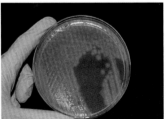

(3)

(4)

DESCRIPTION Gram-negative rod (1)

INFECTIONS
PRIMARY

Head and neck:
  Ear—otitis externa (often referred to as swimmers ear) and otitis media, malignant otitis externa
  Eye—conjunctivitis, keratitis, and other infections
Respiratory: pneumonia
Skin and soft tissue, musculoskeletal:
  Folliculitis—often referred to as hot tub folliculitis
  Ecthyma gangrenosum
  Wound infections
  Osteomyelitis
  Septic arthritis
Systemic: bacteremia
Renal/urinary: UTIs

PATHOGENESIS

Adhesins: pili, capsule
Flagella
Invasins: proteases, hemolysins
Exotoxin: exotoxin A—blocks elongation factor-2 (EF-2) (similar to ● 17, *Corynebacterium diphtheriae* ●)
Biofilm formation
LPS, also called endotoxin—contributes to sepsis

EPIDEMIOLOGY

Inhabitant of soil and water
Transmission:
  Contact with reservoirs, such as water
  Contaminated medical equipment
  Direct contact with infected carrier
Colonizes respiratory tract of individuals with cystic fibrosis
Opportunistic pathogen
Nosocomial pathogen
High risk:
  Malignant otitis externa—diabetics
  Respiratory infections—frequent pathogen of ventilator-associated pneumonia
  Folliculitis—hot tub use
  Wound infections—burn patients

DIAGNOSIS

Culture: aerobic, oxidase positive, lactose negative (2), noncarbohydrate fermenter, metallic sheen (3), grape-like or corn-taco odor; pigment production with pyoverdin is green (4), with pyocyanin is blue, with pyorubin is red

TREATMENT

Piperacillin-tazobactam, ceftazidime, cefepime, meropenem

Explanation 1: *Pseudomonas aeruginosa* is an oxidase-positive, lactose-negative, gram-negative rod. It is the main pathogen of outer ear infections. Infections often arise following swimming and hence are called "swimmer's ear." *P. aeruginosa* has many virulence factors.

Explanation 2: *Pseudomonas aeruginosa* is an oxidase-positive, lactose-negative, gram-negative rod. It is an agent of pneumonia. In hospital-acquired pneumonia, it is associated with ventilators, as in this case. In community-acquired pneumonia, it is associated with cystic fibrosis.

134 *Staphylococcus aureus*

Vignette 1: A 15-year-old girl presents to the emergency department with a 2-day history of fever, chills, myalgia, headache, and watery diarrhea. Her mother states that the symptoms suddenly started, and her daughter seems lethargic and disoriented and is not acting normal. The girl recently started her first menses. Her temperature is 39.3°C (102.7°F), and her blood pressure is 75/60 mm Hg. A diffuse, erythematous, macular rash is present on her extremities and on her palms and soles. Her WBC count is 10.1×10^9/L, and her platelet count is 80×10^9/L. The CSF Gram stain shows no organisms, and the CSF cell count is normal. After 2 days, blood cultures grow gram-positive cocci.

Vignette 2: A 52-year-old man leaves work during the early afternoon with nausea, abdominal cramps, and vomiting. Earlier that day he had consumed several chocolate eclairs at an office party. Several of his coworkers are also experiencing similar symptoms.

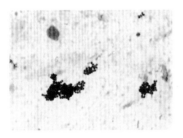

(1)

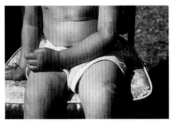

(2) *Source:*
CDC public health library PHIL (phil.cdc.gov) image No. 5155
(http://phil.cdc.gov/phil/details_linked.asp?pid=5155)

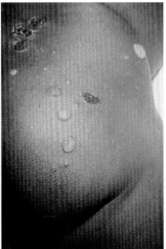

(4) *Source:*
CDC/ Bruno Coignard, M.D.; Jeff Hageman, M.H.S.
CDC public health library PHIL (phil.cdc.gov) image No. 7826
(http://phil.cdc.gov/phil/details_linked.asp?pid=7826)

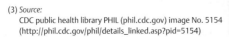

(3) *Source:*
CDC public health library PHIL (phil.cdc.gov) image No. 5154
(http://phil.cdc.gov/phil/details_linked.asp?pid=5154)

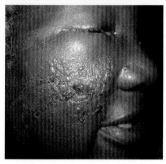

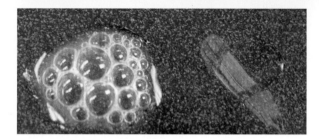

(6) Left, catalase positive. Right, catalase negative.

(5) *Source:* CDC/ Dr. Thomas F. Sellers, Emory University
CDC public health library PHIL (phil.cdc.gov) image
No. 2875
(http://phil.cdc.gov/phil/details_linked.asp?pid=2875)

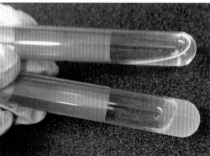

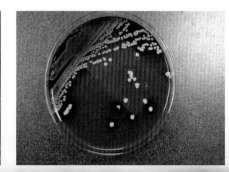

(7) Top, coagulase negative.
Bottom, coagulase positive.

(8)

DESCRIPTION Gram-positive cocci in clusters (1)

INFECTIONS

PRIMARY
Cardiovascular: infective endocarditis (IE)
Gastrointestinal: foodborne illness—nausea and vomiting (short incubation / 1- to 6-hours)
Skin and soft tissue:
    Scalded skin syndrome (SSS)
    Impetigo (described as "honey crusted" lesions) (2,3)
      See also ● 135, *Streptococcus pyogenes* ●
    Folliculitis, furuncle, carbuncle, abscesses (4)
    Cellulitis, erysipelas (5), necrotizing fasciitis
    Surgical-site infections
Musculoskeletal: septic arthritis, osteomyelitis
Renal/urinary: UTIs
Systemic: bacteremia, toxic shock syndrome (TSS)

OTHER
Head and neck:
    Ear—otitis media and externa
    Eye—conjunctivitis
Nervous: meningitis, brain abscesses
Respiratory: sinusitis, epiglottitis, pneumonia (community or hospital acquired)

PATHOGENESIS
Adhesins: capsule, protein A (binds Fc of IgG), coagulase (binds prothrombin), fibronectin binding protein
Exotoxins:
    Enterotoxin—heat stable; stimulates vagus nerve; contributes to foodborne illness
    TSS toxin—superantigen that non-specifically activates T cells
      See also ● 135, *Streptococcus pyogenes* ●
    Exfoliative toxin—cleaves desmoglein; contributes to SSS
    Alpha-toxin (cytotoxin)
    Panton-Valentine leukocidin (PVL)
Tissue enzymes: hyaluronidase, proteases, lipases; facilitate tissue invasion
Resistance to antimicrobials:
    Penicillinase (beta-lactamase)—confers resistance to beta-lactam agents
    mecA gene—mediates resistance to methicillin, penicillins, and related agents

EPIDEMIOLOGY
Normal microbiota of skin and mucous membranes; may colonize nares
Transmission:
    Displacement of endogenous strains
    Direct contact with infected individual or carrier
    Foodborne: ingestion of preformed toxin—commonly associated with potato salad or custard filled pastries, processed meats and salads
High risk:
    IE—most common bacterial pathogen of IE; frequently associated with IV drug use (tricuspid valve frequently involved in IVDU)
    SSS—most common in newborns and children < 5-years-old
    TSS: associated with tampon use
    Meningitis: associated with head trauma
Methicillin-resistant *S. aureus* (MRSA) may be community acquired or nosocomial

DIAGNOSIS
Culture: catalase positive (6), coagulase positive (7), beta-hemolytic on blood agar (8)
Toxin detection for toxin producing strains

TREATMENT   Varies with infection site and clinical setting

Methicillin sensitive *S. aureus* (MSSA)—nafcillin, oxacillin, cefazolin

MRSA—vancomycin, linezolid, daptomycin, ceftaroline

ANIMATION   http://go.thieme.com/microb/Video134.1

Explanation 1: This is a case of toxic shock syndrome caused by toxic shock syndrome toxin-1 (TSST-1) producing strains of *Staphylococcus aureus*. This exotoxin is a superantigen and activates T cells. Superantigens by-pass antigen-presenting cells and directly interact with MHC II. The activation of the T cells results in the release of large amounts of proinflammatory cytokines including IL-1 and -2, IFN-alpha, and TNF-alpha and beta. Most often diagnosis is made based on clinical criteria. The CDC has outlined clinical criteria for toxic shock syndrome and including fever ≥ 38.9°C (102.0°F), hypotension, diffuse erythroderma, desquamation, and involvement of at least three organ systems. Although infections are classically associated with tampon use, most infections are not related to menstruation. Note that blood cultures are only positive in a small percentage of septic shock syndrome cases.

Explanation 2: This man is experiencing food "poisoning" caused by enterotoxin strains of *Staphylococcus aureus*. The enterotoxin stimulates the vagus nerve leading to nausea and vomiting. Watery diarrhea is not common, but may occur in some cases as well. The enterotoxin is heat stable, and can survive both boiling and the stomach acid. Common foods associated with infection include bakery products such as cream-filled pastries, meats, poultry and eggs, milk and dairy products, and salads such as egg, potato, macaroni, and chicken salad. Infections appear rapidly (1 to 6 hours) after ingestion of the toxin, which is preformed, in food.

See also ● 61, *Bacillus cereus* ●

Micro gem: *Streptococcus pyogenes* is the most common bacterial agent of pharyngitis. Other bacterial agents of pharyngitis include ● 17, *Corynebacterium diphtheriae* ● and ● 105, *Neisseria gonorrhoeae* ●. However, it is important to note that viruses are more likely to be implicated in pharyngitis than bacteria.

Vignette: A 7-year-old girl wakes up in the morning complaining of a sore throat. Her temperature at the time is 38.0°C (100.4°F). She stays home from school and refuses to eat all day. Later that evening, when her mother went to check on her, she felt warmer than before and was complaining that her throat hurt so badly she couldn't sleep. Her mother takes her to the urgent care clinic, and her temperature is noted to be 38.9°C (102.0°F). On examination, the girl's throat is severely red with white exudate on both tonsils. Cervical lymphadenopathy is present. A swab of the throat is obtained and sent for culture. The throat culture grows beta-hemolytic, bacitracin-sensitive, gram-positive cocci.

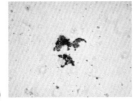

(1)

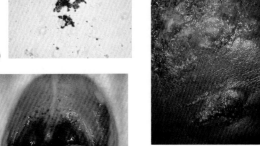

(2) *Source:* CDC/Heinz F. Eichenwald, MD CDC public health library PHIL (phil.cdc.gov) image No. 3185 (http://phil.cdc.gov/phil/details_linked.asp?pid=3185)

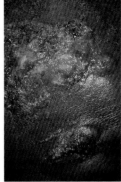

(3) *Source:* CDC/Dr. Thomas F. Sellers; Emory University CDC public health library PHIL (phil.cdc.gov) image No. 14922 (http://phil.cdc.gov/phil/details_linked.asp?pid=14922)

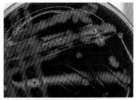

(4) Beta-beta hemolytic.

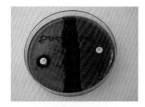

(6) Sensitive (*left*). Resistant (*right*).

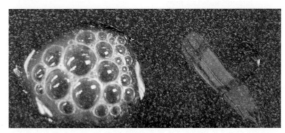

(5) Positive (*left*). Negative (*right*).

DESCRIPTION

Gram-positive cocci in chains (1)
Alternative name: group A streptococcus (GAS)

INFECTIONS

PRIMARY

Head and neck: pharynx—pharyngitis (2)
Skin and soft tissue/musculoskeletal:
  Scarlet fever
  Impetigo ("honey crusted" lesions) (3)
    See also ● 134, *Streptococcus aureus* ●
  Erysipelas
  Cellulitis
  Necrotizing fasciitis, myositis, myonecrosis
Systemic: toxic shock–like syndrome

OTHER

Secondary sequelae
  Head and neck: peritonsillar abscess, sinusitis, mastoiditis
    Ear—otitis media
  Cardiovascular: rheumatic fever
  Kidney: glomerulonephritis (urine often described as "Coca-Cola colored urine")
  Nervous: pediatric autoimmune neuropsychiatric disorder associated with streptococcal infection (PANDAS)

PATHOGENESIS

Immune system escape
  M protein: antiphagocytic
  C5a peptidase: cleaves C5a
Exotoxins: pyrogenic toxins—superantigen activity
  Example: erythrogenic toxin—contributes to scarlet fever

Enzymes
  Streptolysin O and S: lyse RBCs, WBCs, platelets
  Streptokinase: aids in clot dissolution
  Hyaluronidase: degrades hyaluronic acid
  DNAse: cleaves DNA
Immune mediated
  Rheumatic fever: mediated by cross-reactive antibodies (molecular mimicry)
  Glomerulonephritis: mediated by antigen-antibody complexes

EPIDEMIOLOGY

Transmission:
  Pharyngitis: respiratory droplets/secretions
  Skin and soft tissue: direct contact with skin, usually after trauma to skin

DIAGNOSIS

Culture: beta-hemolytic (4), catalase negative (5), bacitracin sensitive (6)
Detection of A carbohydrate
Rapid antigen detection for pharyngitis
Serology: antibody testing—used for post-streptococcal sequelae
  Anti-streptolysin O (ASO)
  Anti-DNAase
Jones criteria: used for the diagnosis of rheumatic fever

TREATMENT

Penicillin; if allergic to penicillin—azithromycin, clindamycin

Explanation: *Streptococcus pyogenes* causes a variety of infections, notably "strep" throat. *S. pyogenes* is a gram-positive coccus in chains and is the most common bacterial agent of pharyngitis. Pharyngitis is self-limiting, but it is important for these infections to be treated due to the secondary immunologic sequelae that may occur, including rheumatic fever and glomerulonephritis.

Micro gem: *S. pneumoniae* is the most common cause of community-acquired bacterial pneumonia and most common cause of meningitis in older adults.

Vignette 1: A 2-year-old boy presents to the emergency department with drainage from the right ear. His mother states that the child has been running a fever and has had a runny nose for the past 2 days. In addition, he has been extremely fussy. At the time of the examination, his temperature is 39.1°C (102.4°F). The drainage from the ear is purulent, and the eardrum has ruptured. A Gram stain from the drainage shows gram-positive diplococci in pairs.

Vignette 2: A previously healthy 77-year-old man is brought to the emergency department with tachypnea and severe chest discomfort. He states that a few days ago he started experiencing chills, a productive cough, and pain in his side. Upon examination his temperature is 38.9°C (102.0°F) and his pulse is 125/min. Chest auscultation demonstrates significant bilateral crackles with expiratory wheezes, and a chest radiograph shows bilateral, diffuse pulmonary infiltrates with effusion. A sputum Gram stain demonstrates the presence of gram-positive diplococci.

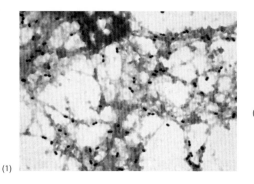

(1)

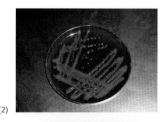

(2)

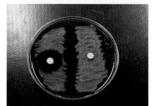

(3) Positive (*left*). Negative (*right*).

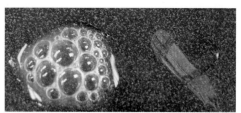

(4) Sensitive (*left*). Resistant (*right*).

DESCRIPTION Gram-positive cocci in pairs (diplococci) and chains (1), lancet-shaped
Alternative name: pneumococcus

INFECTIONS
PRIMARY

Head and neck: sinusitis
   Ear—otitis media
   Eye—conjunctivitis
Nervous: meningitis
Respiratory: pneumonia, acute exacerbation of COPD (*See also* ● 130, *Haemophilus influenzae* ●; ● 16, *Moraxella catarrhalis* ●)
   Pneumonia is usually lobar; sputum often described as rust-colored
Systemic: bacteremia

PATHOGENESIS Capsule: many capsular serotypes
Pneumolysin
IgA protease: destroys IgA
   See also ● 130, *Haemophilus influenzae* ●; ● 105, *Neisseria gonorrhoeae* ●; ● 4, *Neisseria meningitidis* ●

EPIDEMIOLOGY Colonizer of the nasopharynx and some individuals are asymptomatic carriers
Transmission: respiratory droplets/secretions, endogenous translocation
Meningitis most common in older adults and children > 6 months old
High risk:
   Individuals with complement deficiency or antibody defects
   Asplenic individuals
      See also ● 130, *Haemophilus influenzae* ●; ● 4, *Neisseria meningitidis* ●

DIAGNOSIS Culture: alpha-hemolytic (2), catalase negative (3), optochin sensitive (4), bile soluble
Quelling test (used in the past): detection of capsular serotypes
Serology: antigen detection—urine antigen test

PREVENTION Pneumococcal conjugate vaccine (for children < 5-years-old and adults >65-years-old)—currently contains polysaccharide antigens to 13 serotypes
Pneumococcal polysaccharide vaccine (for adults > 65-years-old)—currently contains polysaccharide antigens to 23 serotypes

TREATMENT Depends if isolate is penicillin susceptible or resistant and if a meningeal infection is present
Penicillin-sensitive strains: penicillin G, ceftriaxone, levofloxacin
Penicillin-resistant strains: vancomycin, ceftriaxone, levofloxacin

ANIMATION http://go.thieme.com/microb/Video136.1

Explanation 1 and 2: *Streptococcus pneumoniae* is a gram-positive diplococcus that is lancet shaped. This organism causes a variety of infections including pneumonia (most often consolidation pneumonia) and ear infections. This organism has a capsule and produces several toxic substances including pneumolysin, a pore-forming toxin.

Micro gem: The most common bacterial agents of infective endocarditis are viridans streptococci, ●134, *Staphylococcus aureus* ● (the most common pathogen), ●128, *Enterococcus* ●, and ●126, Coagulase-negative *Staphylococcus* ●. Other bacterial pathogens that may also be involved in infective endocarditis include ● 42, *Bartonella* ●, ●127, *Coxiella burnetti* ●, and members of the HACEK group (see below for individual pathogens).

The HACEK group are slow gram-negative rods that are part of the normal oral microbiota. Because these pathogens often do not grow well in culture infections with these pathogens are often referred to as culture negative endocarditis.

HACEK
*H*aemophilus species
*A*ggregatibacter actinomycetemcomitans
*C*ardiobacterium hominis
*E*ikenella corrodens
*K*ingella kingae

Vignette: A 56-year-old woman presents with fever, chest pain, and painful nodules on her fingers. About 2 weeks ago she had undergone a dental extraction. Her temperature is 38.8°C (101.8°F). Physical exam reveals a murmur, and an echocardiogram shows a small vegetation on her mitral valve. (1)

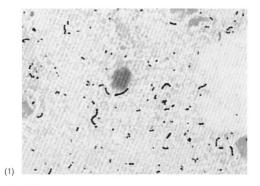

(1)

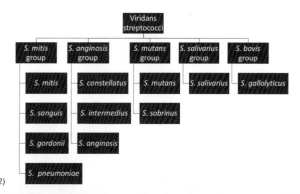

(2)

137 Viridans streptococci

DESCRIPTION
Gram-positive cocci in chains
Viridans streptococci includes *S. anginosus* group, *S. bovis* group, *S. mitis* group, *S. mutans* group, and *S. salivaris* group (2)

INFECTIONS
PRIMARY

S. anginosus group
  Nervous: brain abscess
  Liver: liver abscess
  Respiratory: lung abscess
S. bovis group
  Cardiovascular: infective endocarditis
  Systemic: bacteremia
S. mitis group
  Respiratory: pneumonia
  Systemic: sepsis
S. mutans group
  Oral: dental carries
S. salivaris group
  Cardiovascular: infective endocarditis
  Nervous: meningitis
  Systemic: bacteremia

EPIDEMIOLOGY
Normal microbiota of the oral cavity and GI tract
Transmission: most often due to displacement of endogenous strains
S. bovis group: infections associated with subsequent development of colon cancer
S. mitis group: associated with neutropenia
Infective endocarditis associated with poor dentition or dental manipulation

DIAGNOSIS
Culture: most species are alpha- or gamma-hemolytic; *S. anginosus* may be alpha, beta, or gamma

TREATMENT
Depends on site of infection
Penicillin, vancomycin, ceftriaxone

Explanation: Infective endocarditis may be caused by a number of organisms, including virdans streptococci which is frequently associated with native valve endocarditis. Viridans streptococci includes several organisms and some of these bacteria species are normal microbiota of the oral cavity. Poor dentition and dental manipulation are risk factors for viridans streptococci–mediated infective endocarditis. Viridans streptococci can be displaced from the oral cavity following dental work and seed the bloodstream and subsequently are deposited on cardiac valves. Streptococci are gram-positive cocci in chains.

Vignette: A previously healthy 55-year-old man presents with a 4-day history of fever and painful swelling of his thigh. He lives alone in a wooded mountain area in Eastern California. He has not traveled recently, but reports that he has recently had an infestation of mice in his cabin. His temperature is 38.5°C (101.3°F). On examination, enlargement of the lymph node in his right groin is noted. The fluid from the bubo is aspirated and shows small gram-negative rods.

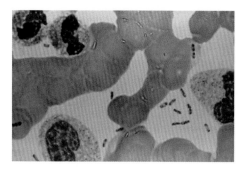

(1) *Source:* CDC public health library PHIL (phil.cdc.gov) image No. 2050
(http://phil.cdc.gov/phil/details_linked.asp?pid=2050)

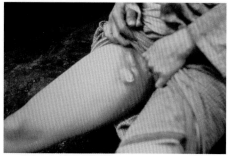

(2) *Source:* CDC public health library PHIL (phil.cdc.gov) image No. 2047
(http://phil.cdc.gov/phil/details_linked.asp?pid=2047)

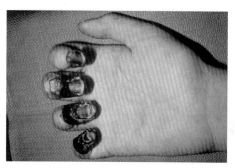

(3) *Source:* CDC/ William Archibald
CDC public health library PHIL (phil.cdc.gov) image No. 1957
(http://phil.cdc.gov/phil/details_linked.asp?pid=1957)

DESCRIPTION

Gram-negative rod or coccobacilli (1); part of *Enterobacteriaceae* family

See also ● 129, *Escherichia coli* ●; ● 103, *Klebsiella granulomatis* ●; ● 131, *Klebsiella pneumoniae* ●; ● 97, *Proteus* ●; ● 47, *Salmonella enterica* serotype typhi and paratyphi ●; ● 70, Nontyphoidal *Salmonella* ●; ● 71, *Shigella* ●; ● 74, *Yersinia enterocolitica* and *pseudotuberculosis* ●

Bipolar staining with Giemsa, Wayson, Wright's stains (1)

Described as "safety pin-like" due to the end of the organisms taking up the stain while the center does not

INFECTIONS
PRIMARY

Plague

Skin and soft tissue/lymphatic: bubonic plague—possible pustule at bite site; bubo formation (2)

Complication: DIC and peripheral gangrene may occur (3)

Respiratory: pneumonic plague

May be primary or secondary (following bubonic plague)

Systemic: septicemic plague

PATHOGENESIS

Endotoxin/LPS: can trigger platelet aggregation and coagulation cascade leading to DIC

Plasminogen activator

Coagulase

Yops protein: assists in immune system evasion

V antigen: intracellular survival

EPIDEMIOLOGY

Zoonotic—reservoirs include rodents, rabbits, squirrels, prairie dogs, domestic/wild cats

Transmission:

Bite of flea: bubonic, septicemic

Contact with infected animal or secretions: bubonic, septicemic

Respiratory droplets (person-to-person): pneumonic

Geographic distribution: in U.S. highest incidence in the southwest

DIAGNOSIS

Culture—only performed at select laboratories

Appropriate safety precautions must be followed when working with this organism

Serology: antibody testing—available from CDC

TREATMENT

Gentamicin, doxycycline

Explanation: This man has bubonic plague caused by *Yersinia pestis*, a gram-negative rod. This pathogen is transmitted by the bite of a flea, contact with contaminated animals, such as mice, or their secretions, or respiratory droplets from an infected individual. In bubonic plaque, swollen and inflamed lymph nodes, known as buboes, are present and are most often seen in the groin and axilla. Other forms of plague include pneumonic and septicemic plague.

Vignette: A 25-year-old woman presents to her physician with painful genital ulcers and dysuria. She also states she has been feeling feverish and has had horrible headaches for the past few days. She recently broke up with her boyfriend of 5 months. Upon examination her temperature is 38.8°C (101.8°F). Inguinal lymphadenopathy is noted, and multiple, shallow, tender vesicular ulcers on the vulva are present. Viral cultures from the ulcers demonstrate the presence of large multinucleated cells.

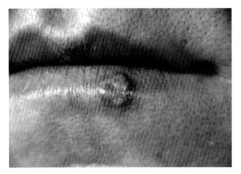

(1) *Source:* CDC/Dr. Herrmann
 CDC public health library PHIL (phil.cdc.gov) image No. 1573
 (http://phil.cdc.gov/phil/details_linked.asp?pid=1573)

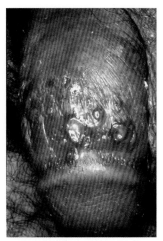

(2) *Source:* CDC/Dr. N.J. Flumara; Dr. Gavin Hart
 CDC public health library PHIL (phil.cdc.gov) image No. 6471
 (http://phil.cdc.gov/phil/details_linked.asp?pid=6471)

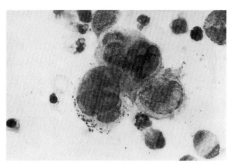

(3) *Source:* CDC/Joe Miller
 CDC public health library PHIL (phil.cdc.gov) image No. 6508
 (http://phil.cdc.gov/phil/details_linked.asp?pid=6508)

139 Herpes simplex virus (HSV)-1 and -2

DESCRIPTION

Taxonomy: Herpesvirus family
See also ● 48, Cytomegalovirus (CMV) ●; ● 51, Epstein-Barr virus (EBV) ●; ● 52, Human herpes virus-6 (HHV-6) ●; ● 117, Varicella-zoster virus ●
Virus properties: double-stranded DNA, enveloped

INFECTIONS

Infections may be primary (first-episode) or recurrent
Mainly HSV-1
    Head and neck:
        Eye—keratoconjunctivitis (recurrent)
        Oral cavity—gingivostomatitis (primary), herpes labialis/ cold sores (recurrent) (1)
    Gastrointestinal: esophagitis
        See also ● 48, Cytomegalovirus (CMV) ●; ● 143, *Candida* species ●
    Nervous: meningitis, encephalitis—most often affect temporal lobe (recurrent)
    Respiratory: pharyngitis (primary)
    Skin and soft tissue: herpetic whitlow—usually on fingers; herpes gladiatorum—usually on arms, face and neck
Mainly HSV-2
    Reproductive: genital herpes—painful vesicular lesions (2); with lymphadenopathy
        See also ● 102, *Haemophilus ducreyi* ●; ● 103, *Klebsiella granulomatis* ●; ● 100, *Chlamydia trachomatis* ●; ● 106, *Treponema pallidum* ●
    Congenital/neonatal: vesicular lesions on skin, eye, and mouth; encephalitis

PATHOGENESIS

TORCH = congenital infections
● 14, *Toxoplasma gondii* ●; **O**ther (● 106, *Treponema pallidum* ●; ● 117, Varicella-zoster virus ●; ● 55, Parvovirus B19 ●); ● 142, **R**ubella virus ●; ● 48, **C**ytomegalovirus (CMV) ●; ● **H**erpes simplex virus ●

Following a primary infection, the virus remains latent in ganglia (HSV-1 in trigeminal; HSV-2 in sacral) and then reactivates resulting in recurrent infections.

EPIDEMIOLOGY

Transmission:
    HSV-1: usually saliva/respiratory secretions
    HSV-2:
        Genital herpes—sexual contact
        Congenital/neonatal—vertical (usually perinatal; but may also be *in utero*)
High risk:
    Herpetic whitlow: associated with healthcare professionals, especially dentist whose hands/fingers may be exposed to oral herpes
    Herpes gladiatorum—associated with wrestlers
    Esophagitis: immunocompromised, especially individuals with AIDS with CD4 T-cells < 100 cells/mm^3
HSV is the most common cause of sporadic encephalitis in the U.S.—may occur in immunocompetent individuals
Recurrence common in immunocompromised, especially in AIDS and transplant recipients

DIAGNOSIS

Viral culture
Serology
    Antigen testing—direct fluorescence antibody (DFA)
    Antibody testing—IgG antibody; IgM not useful
PCR
Microscopy
    Tzanck smear—cells from base of lesion are enlarged and multinucleated (3)
Cowdry type A inclusions—eosinophilic intranuclear bodies from HSV infected cells
Keratitis: slit lamp exam with fluorescein staining—characteristic dendrites seen

TREATMENT

Depends on infection site, immune status, and infection type (primary or reactivation)
Primary genital: acyclovir, valacyclovir famciclovir
Acyclovir-resistant HSV: foscarnet

Explanation: Genital herpes is caused by herpes simplex virus (HSV)-1 and HSV-2, which are double-stranded DNA viruses. In the past, HSV-2 was classically thought as the strain most responsible for genital herpes, but recently HSV-1 has been increasingly implicated as well. The classic presentation of genital herpes is vesicular lesions with an erythematous base (often described as dew drops on rose petals) that evolve into painful, ulcerated lesions and crust when healing, sometimes associated with inguinal lymphadenopathy. HSV infections may present as primary infections or secondary infections. It is important to note that HSV remains latent for life.

Micro gem: Non-polio enteroviruses are the most common cause of viral meningitis.

Vignette 1: A 9-month-old boy presents to the urgent care with fever and vomiting of 4 days' duration. The mother states that he refuses to eat and is irritable. In addition, she states that about 2 weeks prior, the child had a runny nose and ear infection. At the time of examination, the infant's temperature is 39.4°C (102.9°F), and bulging fontanels are noted. The physician hospitalizes the child. CSF is collected and reveals normal glucose and protein levels and an elevated lymphocyte count.

Vignette 2: A 2-year-old boy wakes up crying and his mother notices that he feels warm. She takes his temperature, which is 38.8°C (101.8°F), and administers an anti-pyretic medication. The next morning the boy still has a fever, and the mother notes that his throat is red. She takes the boy to the emergency department. At the time of examination, the boy's temperature is 38.5°C (101.3°F). The physician notes small ulcers on the boy's mouth and tonsils. No rash is present on the boy's body. The mother mentions that the boy attends day care.

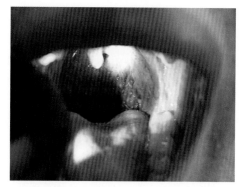

(1) *Source:* By Aphilosophicalmind (own work) [Public domain], via Wikimedia Commons (https://commons.wikimedia.org/wiki/File%3AHerpangina_Virus.JPG)

DESCRIPTION

Taxonomy: Picornavirus family
See also ● 89, Hepatitis A virus ●; ● 8, Poliovirus ●; ● 33, Rhinovirus ●
Virus properties: single-stranded, positive-sense RNA, non-enveloped
Non-polio enteroviruses include group A coxsackie virus, group B coxsackie virus, echovirus, enterovirus
Several serotypes of each virus

INFECTIONS

PRIMARY

Nervous: meningitis, encephalitis—most often Coxsackie B
   Head and neck: herpangina (1) (enanthem)—most often Coxsackie A
   Skin: hand-foot-and-mouth disease (HFMD) (enanthem and exanthem)—most often Coxsackie A

OTHER

Head and neck: eye—acute hemorrhagic conjunctivitis
Cardiovascular: myocarditis, pericarditis—most often Coxsackie B
Respiratory: rhinitis, bronchiolitis, pneumonia
Other: pleurodynia—most often Coxsackie B

EPIDEMIOLOGY

Transmission:
   Fecal-oral
   Contaminated food and water
   Infected oral/respiratory secretions
   Vesicle fluid
   Fomites
Most common infectious agents of aseptic meningitis
Herpangina and HFMD are more common in children.

DIAGNOSIS

Depends on infection type; usually made on clinical findings
Viral culture
Serology: antibody testing
PCR

TREATMENT

Supportive

Explanation 1: Non-polio enteroviruses, especially Coxsackie B viruses, are the most common viral agents involved in aseptic meningitis. These are single-stranded RNA viruses. The main differences in laboratory values between bacterial and viral meningitis is that in bacterial meningitis the CSF glucose is usually low and protein is elevated, with neutrophils being the main cell type observed. This is in contrast to viral meningitis, in which the glucose and protein are most often normal and the main cell types seen are mononuclear cells. Viral meningitis is often referred to as aseptic meningitis because no organisms are isolated on traditional artificial (bacterial) microbiology media.

Explanation 2: This is most likely a case of herpangina caused by Coxsackie A virus. It may present similarly to "strep throat" caused by ● 135, *Streptococcus pyogenes* ●, and patients may present with a painful enanthem. Coxsackie virus is a single-stranded, positive-sense RNA virus that is part of the Enterovirus genera. Coxsackie viruses are also involved in other infections, notably viral meningitis, and hand-foot-and-mouth disease (oral lesions as well as lesions on the hands and feet of young children). Herpangina and hand-foot-and-mouth disease are common infections of young children, and outbreaks often occur in day-care centers.

Vignette: A 31-year-old man is brought to the clinic by his sister because she has noticed that over the past month he has been acting strangely and seems to be more clumsy than normal. The man has previously been diagnosed as HIV positive but has not been compliant with highly active antiretroviral therapy (HAART). The man is confused and not oriented to time or place. Other relevant findings on exam include an ataxic gait and diplopia. The man's current CD4 count is 121/mm³. MRI and biopsy confirm the diagnosis.

DESCRIPTION Taxonomy: Polyoma family; *Polyomavirus* genus
Virus properties: double-stranded DNA, non-enveloped

INFECTIONS
  PRIMARY BK virus
    Kidney: hemorrhagic cystitis, nephritis
  JC virus
    Nervous: progressive multifocal leukoencephalopathy (PML)

PATHOGENESIS JC virus infects oligodendrocytes, which results in demyelination.

EPIDEMIOLOGY Transmission: person-to-person, but exact mechanisms are unclear
BK nephritis associated with kidney transplant
JK virus PML associated with HIV/AIDS

DIAGNOSIS PCR

TREATMENT Supportive.
Although some antiviral agents have been shown to be effective against BK, there is currently no recommended agent for either virus.

Explanation: JC virus is the agent of progressive multifocal leukoencephalopathy (PML), which is mainly associated with AIDS patient with low CD4 counts. The infection may present similarly to toxoplasmosis, herpes encephalitis, and other common infections of AIDS. Common findings of PML include altered mental status, ataxia, motor deficits, and vision impairment. Laboratory analysis such as PCR may aid in diagnosis, as may MRI and biopsy.

Micro gem: TORCH infections are common congenital infections
- 14, **T**oxoplasma gondii
  Other (106, *Treponema pallidum* , 117, Varicella-zoster virus , 55, Parvovirus B19)
- **R**ubella virus
- 48, **C**ytomegalovirus (CMV)
- 139, **H**erpes simplex virus (HSV)-1 and -2

Vignette: A pediatrician examines a newborn in the hospital 12 hours after birth. The baby was born full-term by vaginal delivery. The baby's respiratory rate is elevated, and the physical examination reveals a continuous heart murmur heard best at the upper left sternal border. A chest radiograph demonstrates left atrial and left ventricular enlargement. The ascending aorta is also enlarged, and there is increased pulmonary blood flow. The mother states the pregnancy was uneventful, and her first trimester screen for chromosomal abnormalities was negative. She does not have a history of sexually transmitted infections, and she has never been vaccinated.

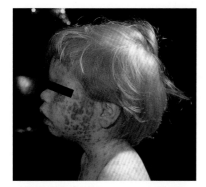

(1) *Source:* CDC public health library PHIL (phil.cdc.gov) image
No. 10145
(http://phil.cdc.gov/phil/details_linked.asp?pid=10145)

142   Rubella virus

DESCRIPTION
Taxonomy: Togavirus family; *Rubivirus* genus
See also ● 10, *Alphavirus* ●
Virus properties: single-stranded, positive-sense RNA, enveloped

INFECTIONS
PRIMARY
Rubella, also called German measles
Most often subclinical
Post-natal
Systemic: prodrome—constitutional symptoms
Skin: exanthem—maculopapular rash (1); starts at face and spreads downward
Head and neck: oral cavity—enanthem (Forchheimer spots) may be present on soft palate
Congenital:
Head and neck: ear—hearing loss; eye—cataracts
Cardiovascular: patent ductus arteriosus, pulmonary artery hypoplasia
Skin: petechial rash ("blueberry muffin" rash)

OTHER
Complications in adults
Musculoskeletal: arthritis

EPIDEMIOLOGY
Transmission: respiratory droplets, vertical (*in utero*)

DIAGNOSIS
Serology: antibody testing
PCR
Viral culture

PREVENTION
Vaccine: live, attenuated vaccine

TREATMENT
Supportive

Explanation: Because this mother has never been vaccinated, the most likely pathogen in this case is rubella virus. This pathogen is part of the TORCH group, which is an acronym for perinatal/congenital pathogens: *Toxoplasma gondii*; Other (*Treponema pallidum*/syphilis; varicella-zoster virus; parvovirus B19); Rubella virus; Cytomegalovirus; Herpes simplex virus. Features of congenital rubella include intrauterine growth restriction, hearing loss, cataracts, cardiac abnormalities such as patent ductus arteriosus and pulmonary artery hypoplasia, neurologic issues, and a petechial rash ("blueberry muffin" rash).

Vignette 1: A mother brings her 2-week-old boy to the pediatrician because of a white substance in his mouth. She states that the baby is more fussy than normal, and, although he is feeding, he seems to be eating less. The infant was born at 34½ weeks and the birth was uncomplicated. The baby is exclusively breast-fed, and the mother complains of mammary pain. The infant's temperature is 36.4°C (97.5°F), and on physical examination a thick, white plaque on the buccal mucosa, palate, and tongue is seen. The white substance is easily scraped off of the tongue using a tongue blade.

Vignette 2: A 25-year old woman visits her primary care physician with vaginal itchiness and discharge of 3 days' duration. She takes oral contraceptives. A pelvic exam demonstrates vulvar and mucosal edema and erythema. The discharge is thick, white, and clumpy. A KOH preparation from the discharge reveals the presence of budding yeast and hyphae.

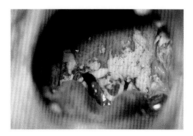
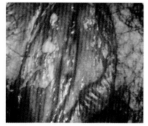
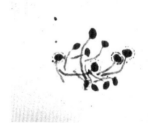
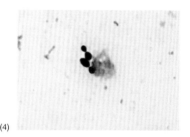

(1) *Source:* CDC public health library PHIL (phil.cdc.gov) image No. 1217 (http://phil.cdc.gov/phil/details_linked.asp?pid=1217)

(2) *Source:* CDC/Susan Lindsley CDC public health library PHIL (phil.cdc.gov) image No. 15679 (http://phil.cdc.gov/phil/details_linked.asp?pid=15679)

(3) *Source:* CDC/Dr. Lucille K. Georg CDC public health library PHIL (phil.cdc.gov) image No. 1214 (http://phil.cdc.gov/phil/details_linked.asp?pid=1214)

(4)

(5)

143 *Candida albicans*

DESCRIPTION
Yeast, pseudohyphae and (true) hyphae
Other clinically significant species include *C. glabrata*, *C. krusei*, *C. parapsilosis*, *C. tropicalis*

INFECTIONS
PRIMARY
Localized mucosal or invasive/disseminated infections
Localized mucosal
  Head and neck: oral cavity—oropharyngeal candidiasis (also called thrush) (1)
  Gastrointestinal: esophagitis
    See also ● 48, Cytomegalovirus (CMV) ●; ● 139, Herpes simplex virus (HSV)-1 and -2 ●
  Reproductive: vulvovaginitis (2)—pruritus, thick, white discharge (often described as "cottage-cheese-like") normal vaginal pH, WBCs present
    See also ● 108, *Trichomonas vaginalis* ●
  Skin and soft tissue: diaper dermatitis, balanitis, intertrigo
  Other: chronic mucocutaneous candidiasis
Invasive/disseminated
  Cardiovascular: endocarditis, pericarditis
  Gastrointestinal: peritonitis
  Nervous: meningitis
  Musculoskeletal: osteomyelitis, septic arthritis
  Renal/urinary: UTIs
  Respiratory: empyema, pneumonia
  Systemic: fungemia

PATHOGENESIS
C. albicans: morphogenesis (ability to transition from yeast to hyphae)—hyphae facilitate invasion

EPIDEMIOLOGY
Many *Candida* species are part of the normal microbiota; *C. albicans* colonize skin and mucosa of vagina, and GI tract.
Transmission: most often from displacement of endogenous strains
Opportunistic pathogen
Risk factors:
  Immunocompromised: especially malignancies, post-transplant, neutropenia, HIV

Oropharyngeal: neonates, immunocompromised
Esophagitis: AIDS, especially with CD4 T-cells < 100 cells/mm^3
Vulvovaginitis: oral contraceptives, increased estrogen, antibiotics
Intertrigo: diabetes mellitus, obesity
Chronic mucocutaneous candidiasis: cell-mediated immune deficiency
Endocarditis: IV drug users, prosthetic valve
Meningitis: ventriculoperitoneal (VP) shunt, CNS surgical procedures

DIAGNOSIS
Fungal culture: growth on Sabouraud dextrose agar
Microscopy: KOH preparation
  C. albicans: germ tube positive (3), budding yeast (4), pseudo-hyphae or hyphae may be seen in tissue (5)
Serology: antigen detection—beta-D-glucan is part of fungal cell wall; not specific for *C. albicans*

TREATMENT
Depends on infecting species, infection site, localized or disseminated infection, age and immune status
Fluconazole, amphotericin B, caspofungin

Explanation 1: This is a case of oropharyngeal candidiasis or thrush. Thrush is most often seen in infants (especially premature infants), immunocompromised adults, and denture wearers. A simple physical exam maneuver to distinguish thrush from other white oral plaques is to scrape the tongue with a tongue blade; white plaque from *Candida* will easily scrape off. In this case the mother's breast may have been infected with *Candida* (mastitis), leading to thrush in the baby. *Candida*, a yeast, is part of the normal microbiota, but may also cause mucocutaneous, systemic, and invasive infections. *C. albicans* is the most notable *Candida* species.

Explanation 2: The typical manifestations of *Candida* vulvovaginitis include vaginal pruritus and irritation. Although the vaginal discharge when infected with *Candida* is very distinct, discharge is not always present. If present, it is usually thick and white (often described as cottage-cheese or curd-like). With vaginitis, the vaginal mucosa is inflamed, and vaginal discharge will demonstrate the presence of white blood cells. The vaginal pH is most often normal. A KOH preparation may be used to better visualize the yeast and hyphal elements

Vignette: A 3-year-old girl presents with a stomachache, fever, and lack of appetite. Her mother states they have been spending a lot of time at the neighborhood playground, and that the sandbox is the child's favorite activity during their visits. The mother also mentions that the child often puts sand in her mouth. The girl's temperature is 38.1°C (100.6°F), and the physical exam reveals hepatosplenomegaly. A CBC shows elevated WBCs with a marked increase in eosinophils. CT shows lesions in the liver. The stool O&P test is negative, but serological tests confirm the diagnosis.

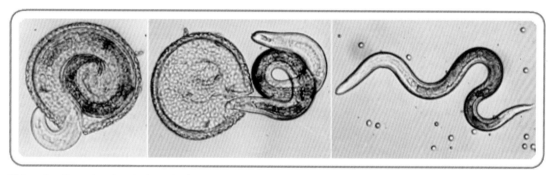

(1) *Source:* http://www.cdc.gov/parasites/toxocariasis/

DESCRIPTION
Nemathelminth / roundworms
Clinically significant morphological forms: ova (eggs), adult worms
Clinically significant species: *T. cati, T. canis*

INFECTIONS
PRIMARY

Multi-organ system: visceral larva migrans—larvae (1) may migrate to any organ
 Common migration locations: liver, lungs, eye
Head and neck: eye—ocular larva migrans; ocular lesions

LIFE CYCLE
Cats (*T. cati*) or dogs (*T. canis*) release eggs (ova) in stool; humans ingest ova in dirt; eggs hatch and form larvae; larvae migrate to various organs
Humans are accidental hosts—larvae do not develop into adults in humans

EPIDEMIOLOGY
Transmission: fecal-oral—ingestion of ova, which may be in the soil or ingestion of undercooked meat with larval form
High risk: young children

DIAGNOSIS
Serology: antibody testing
CBC: eosinophilia

TREATMENT
Depends on infection type and severity of infection
Ocular: supportive
Visceral (severe infections): albendazole

Explanation: Visceral larval migrans is caused by the nematode *Toxocara canis* or less commonly *Toxocara cati*. Infections most often occur following ingestion of the ova, which may be found in dirt, especially dirt contaminated with dog or cat feces. Following ingestion, the ova hatch into larvae, and the larvae migrate to various organs and ultimately induce an inflammatory response. Most often visceral larval migrans is seen in young children and may manifest as hepatitis or pneumonitis. Eosinophilia and hypergammaglobinemia are key features of infection.

Appendix

A1. GRAM STAIN REACTIONS FOR SELECT CLINICALLY SIGNIFICANT BACTERIA

Gram-positive cocci	Gram-positive bacilli	Gram-negative cocci	Gram-negative bacilli	Gram-negative coccobacilli	Organisms that Gram stain poorly

Chains
Enterococcus
Streptococcus
 	
Chains and Pairs
Streptococcus
   pneumoniae
 	
Clusters
Staphylococcus
	Bacillus
	Clostridium
	Erysipelothrix
	Gardnerella
	Lactobacillus
	Listeria monocytogenes
	Propionibacterium acnes
	
	Branching
	Actinomyces
	Nocardia (also modified
	  acid fast)
	
	Palisading, Pleomorphic
	Corynebacterium diphtheriae
		Moraxella
		
		Pairs
		Neisseria
			Curved
			Campylobacter
			Helicobacter
			Vibrio
			
			Aerobes
			Bartonella
			Citrobacter
			Enterobacter
			Escherichia coli
			Legionella
			Klebsiella
			Proteus
			Pseudomonas
			Salmonella
			Serratia
			Shigella
			Yersinia
			
			Anaerobes
			Bacteroides
			Fusobacterium
				Bordetella pertussis
				Brucella
				Coxiella
				Francisella
				Haemophilus
				Pasturella
					Spirochetes
					Borrelia
					Leptospira
					Treponema
					
					Other
					Chlamydia / Chlamydophila
					Mycobacterium
					Mycoplasma
					Anaplasma
					Ehrlichia
					Rickettsia
					Ureaplasma

Media	Purpose	Comments
Blood alpha beta gamma Figure 1. Hemolysis on Blood Agar	Enriched, non-selective media that supports the growth of a wide variety of bacteria and some fungi	Enriched with red blood cells; some bacteria may hemolyze red blood cells leading to hemolysis; Alpha hemolysis—partial hemolysis; beta hemolysis—complete hemolysis; gamma hemolysis—no hemolysis
Chocolate	Enriched, non-selective media that supports growth of a wide variety of bacteria and some fungi; supports the growth of *Haemophilus* and *Neisseria*	Enriched with X (hemin) and V (NAD) factors
Eosin Methylene Blue (EMB) Figure 2. *E. coli* on EMB Agar	Selective for enteric gram-negative bacilli Differential for lactose reactions	*E. coli* produces a green metallic sheen

Media	Purpose	Comments
Hektoen Uninoculated plate Lactose positive Lactose negative Lactose negative, H₂S positive Figure 3. Hektoen Agar	Selective for enteric gram-negative bacilli Differential for lactose reactions and hydrogen sulfide (H$_2$S)	Lactose positive = orange/yellow; Lactose negative = clear/colorless H$_2$S positive = black colonies; H$_2$S negative = green colonies
MacConkey Lactose positive Lactose negative Figure 4. MacConkey Agar, lactose fermentation	Selective for enteric gram-negative bacilli Differential for lactose reactions	Contains bile salts and crystal violet to prevent the growth of gram-positive organisms Lactose positive = pink/red; Lactose negative = clear/colorless

Media	Purpose	Comments
MacConkey with Sorbitol Sorbitol positive Sorbitol negative Figure 5. MacConkey Agar with sorbitol	Selective for enteric gram-negative bacilli Differential for enterohemorrhagic *E. coli* (a.k.a. EHEC or *E. coli* O157:H7)	Sorbitol positive = pink/red; Sorbitol negative = clear/colorless
Thiosulfate citrate bile salts sucrose (TCBS)	Selective for *Vibrio* Differential for sucrose reactions	Sucrose positive = yellow; Sucrose negative = green
Thayer-Martin	Selective for pathogenic *Neisseria*	
Regan-Lowe	Selective for *Bordetella pertussis*	
Bordet-Gengou	Selective for *Bordetella pertussis*	
Buffered Charcoal Yeast Extract (BCYE)	Selective for *Legionella*	
Cystine tellurite	Selective for *Corynebacterium diphtheriae*	
Loefflers	Selective for *Corynebacterium diphtheriae*	
Lowenstein-Jensen	Selective for *Mycobacterium*	

A3. CLINICALLY SIGNIFICANT ANAEROBES

Gram Stain	Infections / Organ Systems						
	Nervous system	GI	Intra-abdominal	Oral Cavity, Neck and Respiratory Tract	Reproductive (female genital tract)	Systemic	Skin and Soft Tissue / Wound
GPR	*Actinomyces* *C. botulinum* *C. tetani*	*C. difficile*		*Actinomyces*	*Actinomyces* *Mobilluncus*		*C. botulinum* *C. perfringens* *Proprionibacterium*
GPC	*Peptostreptococcus*		*Peptostreptococcus*	*Peptostreptococcus*	*Peptostreptococcus*		*Peptostreptococcus*
GNR	*Prevotella* *Porphyromonas* *Fusobacterium*	*B. fragilis*	*B. fragilis* *Prevotella* *Fusobacterium*	*Bacteroides* non *fragilis* *Eikenella* *Fusobacterium* *Prevotella* *Porphyromonas*	*Prevotella*	*B. fragilis*	*B. fragilis*
GNC				*Veillonella*			

A4. COMPARISON OF *ESCHERICHIA COLI* STRAINS

	Primary Infection	Manifestation	Pathogenesis
EAEC	Traveler's diarrhea	Watery diarrhea	Tight adherence Toxin—increases cGMP
EPEC	Infant diarrhea in resource-limited countries	Watery diarrhea	Firm / intimate attachment to enterocyte / pedestal formation
EHEC	Diarrhea	Watery diarrhea that develops into bloody diarrhea	Shiga-like toxin that prevents protein synthesis
EIEC	Diarrhea mainly in resource-limited countries	Dysentery	Invasion of enterocyte

ETEC	Traveler's diarrhea
	Infant diarrhea in resource-limited countries
		Watery diarrhea	Heat-labile toxin
			  LT—increases cAMP
			Heat-stable toxin
			  ST—increases cGMP

A5. SUMMARY OF CLINICALLY SIGNIFICANT VIRUSES

Virus	Family	Genome	Envelope	Disease/Clinical Signs
Herpes simplex virus-1 (HSV-1) (HHV-1)	Herpesvirus	ds-DNA	Yes	• Vesicular orolabial and genital lesions • Meningoencephalitis • Keratitis (classically with dendritic ulcers)
Herpes simplex virus-2 (HSV-2) (HHV-2)	Herpesvirus	ds-DNA	Yes	• Vesicular genital lesions • Meningoencephalitis, incl. neonates after vaginal delivery
Varicella-Zoster virus (HHV-3)	Herpesvirus	ds-DNA	Yes	• Varicella or "chickenpox" • Herpes zoster of "shingles;" may be complicated by post-herpetic neuralgia
Epstein-Barr virus (HHV-4)	Herpesvirus	ds-DNA	Yes	• Infectious mononucleosis • EBV-associated lymphoproliferative diseases: ○ Burkitt lymphoma ○ Nasopharyngeal Ca. ○ Post-transplant lymphoproliferative disorder
Cytomegalovirus (HHV-5)	Herpesvirus	ds-DNA	Yes	• Infectious mononucleosis • Retinitis • Pneumonitis • Esophagitis • Hepatitis • Gastroenteritis • Congenital CMV syndrome
Human herpes virus-6 (HHV-6)	Herpesvirus	ds-DNA	Yes	• Roseola infantum or "Sixth disease"
Human herpes virus-8 (HHV-8)	Herpesvirus	ds-DNA	Yes	• Kaposi sarcoma (classically in AIDS)
Adenovirus	Adenovirus	ds-DNA	No	• Conjunctivitis • Gastroenteritis • Genitourinary infection • Respiratory infection

Red= DNA virus
Blue = RNA virus

Virus	Family	Genome	Envelope	Disease/Clinical Signs
BK virus JC virus	Polyomavirus	ds-DNA	No	• BK: Polyomavirus nephropathy • JC: Progressive multifocal leukoencephalopathy
Human papillomavirus (HPV)	Papillomavirus	ds-DNA	No	• Condylomata acuminate or "genital warts" (low risk HPV: 6, 11) • Cervical Ca. (high risk HPV: 16, 18, 31, 33) • Head and neck papilloma and squamous cell Ca.
Molluscum contagiosum virus	Poxvirus	ds-DNA	Yes	• Molluscum contagiosum (pink/white papules with characteristic central umbilications)
Variola (smallpox) virus	Poxvirus	ds-DNA	Yes	• Smallpox; officially eradicated in 1980
Parvovirus B19	Parvovirus	ss-DNA	No	• Erythema infectiosum or "Fifth disease" • Hydrops fetalis if *in utero* infection • Aplastic crisis in sickle cell disease
Hepatitis A virus (HAV)	Picornavirus	(+) ss-RNA	No	• Self-limited acute hepatitis • Fecal-oral transmission
Hepatitis B virus (HBV)	Hepadnavirus	Partial ds-DNA, circular genome	Yes	• Acute, fulminant, and/or chronic hepatitis • May cause cirrhosis and hepatocellular Ca. • Parenteral transmission
Hepatitis C virus (HCV)	Flavivirus	(+) ss-RNA	Yes	• Chronic hepatitis • May cause cirrhosis and hepatocellular Ca. • Parenteral transmission
Hepatitis D virus (HDV)	Deltavirus	(−) ss-RNA	Yes	• Requires HBV for infection • Super-infection has worse prognosis than co-infection • Parenteral transmission
Hepatitis E virus (HEV)	Hepevirus	(+) ss-RNA	No	• Self-limited acute hepatitis • Fecal-oral transmission • 20% mortality rate in pregnant women

Red= DNA virus
Blue = RNA virus

Virus	Family	Genome	Envelope	Disease/Clinical Signs
Coxsackie virus (a non-polio enterovirus)	Picornavirus	(+) ss-RNA	No	• Hand-Foot-Mouth Disease and herpangina • Myocarditis, pericarditis • Aseptic meningitis
Echovirus (a non-polio enterovirus)	Picornavirus	(+) ss-RNA	No	• Carditis • Aseptic meningitis
Polio virus (an enterovirus)	Picornavirus	(+) ss-RNA	No	• Poliomyelitis
Rhinovirus	Picornavirus	(+) ss-RNA	No	• Upper respiratory tract infection of the "common cold"
Norovirus	Calicivirus	(+) ss-RNA	No	• Gastroenteritis
Human immunodeficiency virus (HIV)	Retrovirus	(+) ss-RNA	Yes	• Acquired Immunodeficiency Syndrome (AIDS)
Human T-cell lymphotropic virus (HTLV)	Retrovirus	(+) ss-RNA	Yes	• T-cell leukemia and lymphoma
Human coronavirus	Coronavirus	(+) ss-RNA	Yes	• Respiratory infection: common cold
Severe Acute Respiratory Syndrome coronavirus (SARS-CoV)	Coronavirus	(+) ss-RNA	Yes	• Respiratory infection: SARS
Influenza viruses A,B,C	Orthomyxovirus	(−) ss-RNA Segmented genome	Yes	• Respiratory infection: influenza • May be complicated by secondary *Staphylococcus aureus* bacterial pneumonia
Measles virus	Paramyxovirus	(−) ss-RNA	Yes	• Measles
Mumps virus	Paramyxovirus	(−) ss-RNA	Yes	• Mumps: may cause parotitis, orchitis, pancreatitis
Parainfluenza virus	Paramyxovirus	(−) ss-RNA	Yes	• Laryngotracheobronchitis or "croup" in young children
Respiratory syncytial virus (RSV)	Paramyxovirus	(−) ss-RNA	Yes	• Respiratory infection: bronchiolitis is babies
Rubella virus	Togavirus	(+) ss-RNA	Yes	• Rubella in kids/adults • Congenital rubella syndrome

Red= DNA virus
Blue = RNA virus

Virus	Family	Genome	Envelope	Disease/Clinical Signs
Alphavirus 　Chikungunya	Togavirus	(+) ss-RNA	Yes	• Febrile illness
Alphavirus 　Eastern Equine Encephalitis 　Western Equine Encephalitis 　Venezuelan Equine Encephalitis	Togavirus	(+) ss-RNA	Yes	• Encephalitis
Dengue virus	Flavivirus	(+) ss-RNA	Yes	• Hemorrhagic and "break-bone" fever
West Nile virus	Flavivirus	(+) ss-RNA	Yes	• Flu-like syndrome • Meningoencephalitis
Yellow fever virus	Flavivirus	(+) ss-RNA	Yes	• Hemorrhagic fever
Zika virus	Flavivirus	(+) ss-RNA	Yes	• Zika fever
Ebola virus Marburg virus	Filovirus	(−) ss-RNA	Yes	• Hemorrhagic fever
Hantavirus	Bunyavirus	(−) ss-RNA	Yes	• Hemorrhagic fever
California encephalitis virus Lacrosse virus	Bunyavirus	(−) ss-RNA	Yes	• Encephalitis
Rabies virus	Rhabdovirus	(−) ss-RNA	Yes	• Rabies
Rotavirus	Reovirus	ds-RNA	No	• Gastroenteritis
Colorado tick virus	Reovirus	ds-RNA	No	• Febrile illness
Lassa virus	Arenavirus	Ambisense RNA	Yes	• Febrile illness; possible hemorrhagic fever

Red= DNA virus
Blue = RNA virus

A6. VIRAL HEPATITIS SUMMARY TABLE

	Hepatitis A virus (HAV)	Hepatitis B virus (HBV)	Hepatitis C virus (HCV)	Hepatitis D virus (HDV)	Hepatitis E virus (HEV)
Common name	Infectious	Serum	Non-A, Non B Posttransfusion	Delta agent	Enteric Non-A, Non-B
Virus properties	Picornavirus SS +RNA	Hepadnavirus DS DNA	Flavivirus SS +RNA	Incomplete virion RNA	Hepevirus SS +RNA
Transmission	Fecal-oral	Body fluids Blood, semen, other fluids Vertical	Primary: contaminated blood Other: sexual, vertical	Needs HBV to replicate; see HBV	Fecal-oral
Average incubation (days)	28	120	45	See HBV	40
Chronicity	No	Yes	Yes	Yes	No
Long-term sequelae of chronic infections	None	Cirrhosis, liver failure, hepatocellular carcinoma	Cirrhosis, hepatocellular carcinoma	See HBV	None
Serology	Acute: IgM anti-HAV Convalescent: IgG anti-HAV Past infection/immunity: total anti-HAV	IgM anti-HBc: acute HBsAg: acute; chronic (> 6 months) Total anti-HBc: acute, chronic, resolved Anti-HBs: recovery/immunity	Cannot distinguish acute from chronic Anti-HCV HCV RNA	Anti-HDV—present in co-infections and superinfections	Acute: IgM anti-HEV Late acute and convalescent: IgG anti-HEV
Vaccination	Inactivated	Recombinant	None	None	None
Antimicrobial	None	Chronic: entecavir, telbivudine, tenofovir	Sofosbuvir, daclatasvir, ledipasvir with or without ribavirin	See HBV	None

Abbreviations: DS, double stranded; HBc, hepatitis B core; HBsAg, hepatitis B surface antigen; Ig, immunoglobulin; SS, single stranded.

A7.   PARASITE FLOW CHART: PROTOZOA

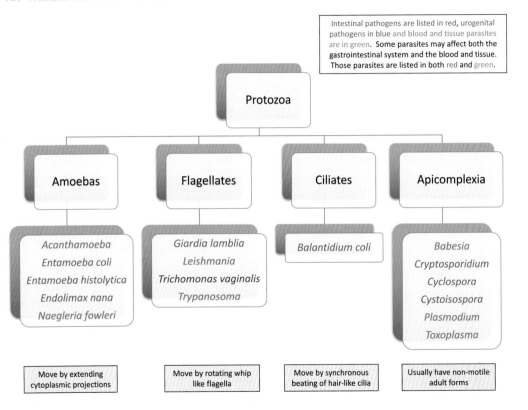

Intestinal pathogens are listed in red, urogenital pathogens in blue and blood and tissue parasites are in green. Some parasites may affect both the gastrointestinal system and the blood and tissue. Those parasites are listed in both red and green.

Protozoa

Amoebas

Acanthamoeba
Entamoeba coli
Entamoeba histolytica
Endolimax nana
Naegleria fowleri

Move by extending cytoplasmic projections

Flagellates

Giardia lamblia
Leishmania
Trichomonas vaginalis
Trypanosoma

Move by rotating whip like flagella

Ciliates

Balantidium coli

Move by synchronous beating of hair-like cilia

Apicomplexia

Babesia
Cryptosporidium
Cyclospora
Cystoisospora
Plasmodium
Toxoplasma

Usually have non-motile adult forms

A8. PARASITE FLOW CHART: WORMS

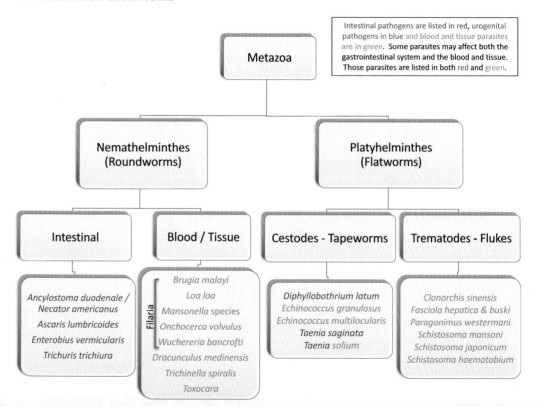

Metazoa

Intestinal pathogens are listed in red, urogenital pathogens in blue and blood and tissue parasites are in green. Some parasites may affect both the gastrointestinal system and the blood and tissue. Those parasites are listed in both red and green.

Nemathelminthes (Roundworms)

Platyhelminthes (Flatworms)

Intestinal

Blood / Tissue

Cestodes - Tapeworms

Trematodes - Flukes

Ancylostoma duodenale / Necator americanus
Ascaris lumbricoides
Enterobius vermicularis
Trichuris trichiura

Filaria
Brugia malayi
Loa loa
Mansonella species
Onchocerca volvulus
Wuchereria bancrofti
Dracunculus medinensis
Trichinella spiralis
Toxocara

Diphyllobothrium latum
Echinococcus granulosus
Echinococcus multilocularis
Taenia saginata
Taenia solium

Clonorchis sinensis
Fasciola hepatica & buski
Paragonimus westermani
Schistosoma mansoni
Schistosoma japonicum
Schistosoma haematobium

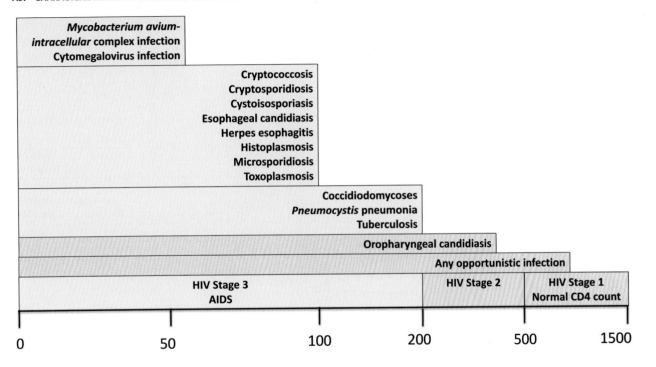

CD4 T-Cell Count

A10. COMPARISON OF GENITAL ULCER DISEASE

Feature	Genital Herpes	Chancroid	Syphilis	LGV	Granuloma Inguinale / Donovanosis
Causative agent	*Herpes simplex virus* (most often type 2)	*Haemophilus ducreyi*	*Treponema pallidum*	*Chlamydia trachomatis* L1, L2, L3	*Klebsiella granulomatis*
Typical lesion	Early on—vesicles • Erythematous Later—ulcer • Shallow • Raised edges	Ulcer • Purulent base • Non-indurated • Ragged edges	Ulcer *I* chancre • Indurated • Demarcated edges	Early on—papule Later—ulcer • Small • Shallow	Ulcer • Highly vascular "beefy red"
Painful or Painless	Painful	Painful	Painless	Painless	Painless
Number of lesions	Multiple	Usually multiple	Usually singular	Usually singular	Variable
Inguinal lymphadenopathy	Yes	Yes buboes	Yes in late 1° syphils	Yes-painful in 2° LGV buboes	Not usually pseudobuboes
Constitutional symptoms	Yes	No	Yes in 2° syphilis	Yes in 2° LGV	No

A11. VAGINITIS/VAGINOSIS DIFFERENTIATION

	Normal	Bacterial Vaginosis	Candidiasis	Trichomoniasis
Symptom presentation		Odor, discharge, itch	Itch, discomfort, dysuria, thick discharge	Itch, discharge, ~70% asymptomatic
Vaginal discharge	Clear to white	Homogenous, adherent, thin, milky white; malodorous "foul fishy"	Thick, clumpy, white "cottage cheese"	Frothy, gray or yellow-green; malodorous
Clinical findings			Inflammation and erythema	Cervical petechiae "strawberry cervix"
Vaginal pH	3.8 - 4.2	> 4.5	Usually ≤ 4.5	> 4.5
KOH "whiff" test	Negative	Positive	Negative	Often positive
NaCl wet mount	Lacto-bacilli	Clue cells (≥ 20%), no/few WBCs	Few to many WBCs	Motile flagellated protozoa, many WBCs
KOH wet mount			Pseudohyphae or spores if non-*albicans* species	

Credit: CDC Vaginitis Curriculum

A12. VECTOR-BORNE INFECTIONS

	Mosquito	Tick	Flea	Mite	Lice	Sandfly
Bacteria		• Tularemia (*Francisella tularensis*) • Recurrent fever (*Borrelia hermsii* and other non *B. recurrentis* species) • Human Granulocytic Anaplasmosis (HGA) (*Anaplasma*) • Human Monocytic Ehrlichiosis (HME) (*Ehrlichia*) • Lyme disease (*Borrelia burgdorferi*) • Rocky Mountain spotted fever (*Rickettsia rickettsii*; RMSF)	• Cat-scratch fever (*Bartonella henselae*) • Plague (*Yersinia pestis*) • Murine (endemic) typhus (*Rickettsia typhi*)	• Rickettsiapox (*Rickettsia akari*) • Scrub typhus (*Orientia tsutsugamushi*)	• Trench fever & bacillary angiomatosis (*Bartonella quintana*) • Relapsing fever (*Borrelia recurrentis*) • Epidemic typhus (*Rickettsia prowazekii*)	• Oroya fever; also called Carrion's disease (*Bartonella bacilliformis*)
Virus	• Chikungunya • Dengue • Eastern, Western & Venezuelan equine encephalitis • Japanese encephalitis • St. Louis encephalitis • West Nile • Yellow fever • Zika	• Colorado tick virus				

	Mosquito	Tick	Flea	Mite	Lice	Sandfly
Parasite	• Lymphadenitis (*Wuchereria bancrofti* & *Brugia malayi*) • Malaria (*Plasmodium*)	• Babesiosis (*Babesia*)				• Leishmaniasis (*Leishmania*)

OTHER

Black fly
• River blindness—(*Onchocerca volvulus*)

Deerfly also called mango fly
• Loaiasis (*Loa loa*)

Reduviid bug also called triatome and kissing bug
• Chagas disease (*Trypanosoma cruzi*)

Tsetse fly
• African sleeping sickness (*Trypanosoma brucei* subsp. gambiense & rhodensiense)

COLOR KEY

Pink = Gram-negative
Green = virus
Orange = parasite
Gray = bacteria that do not Gram stain well